EDITED BY
VINI LANDER, KAVYTA KAY AND
TIFFANY R. HOLLOMAN

COVID-19 AND RACISM

Counter-Stories of Colliding Pandemics

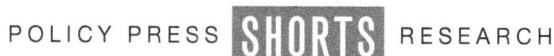

First published in Great Britain in 2023 by

Policy Press, an imprint of
Bristol University Press
University of Bristol
1–9 Old Park Hill
Bristol
BS2 8BB
UK
t: +44 (0)117 374 6645
e: bup-info@bristol.ac.uk

Details of international sales and distribution partners are available at
policy.bristoluniversitypress.co.uk

© Bristol University Press 2023

British Library Cataloguing in Publication Data
A catalogue record for this book is available from the British Library

ISBN 978-1-4473-6673-7 hardcover
ISBN 978-1-4473-6674-4 ePub
ISBN 978-1-4473-6675-1 ePdf

The right of Vini Lander, Kavyta Kay and Tiffany R. Holloman to be identified as editors of this work has been asserted by them in accordance with the Copyright, Designs and Patents Act 1988.

All rights reserved: no part of this publication may be reproduced, stored in a retrieval system, or transmitted in any form or by any means, electronic, mechanical, photocopying, recording, or otherwise without the prior permission of Bristol University Press.

Every reasonable effort has been made to obtain permission to reproduce copyrighted material. If, however, anyone knows of an oversight, please contact the publisher.

The statements and opinions contained within this publication are solely those of the editors and contributors and not of the University of Bristol or Bristol University Press. The University of Bristol and Bristol University Press disclaim responsibility for any injury to persons or property resulting from any material published in this publication.

Bristol University Press and Policy Press work to counter discrimination on grounds of gender, race, disability, age and sexuality.

Cover design: Dave Worth
Front cover image: Stocksy/ZHPH Production and alamy/Artulina1
Bristol University Press and Policy Press use environmentally responsible print partners.
Printed and bound in Great Britain by CPI Group (UK) Ltd, Croydon, CR0 4YY

Contents

Notes on contributors		v
Acknowledgements		x
Introduction: The long road ahead		1
one	BLAME the BAME *Javeria Shah*	10
two	COVID-1984: wake MBE up when Black Lives Matter *Tré Ventour-Griffiths*	14
three	Black vaccination reticence: HBCUs, the Flexner Report and COVID-19 *LaTonia A. Siler-Holloman and Tiffany R. Holloman*	37
four	Pregnancy, pandemic and protest: critical reflections of a Black millennial mother *Sharon Anyiam*	59
five	It's alive! The resurrection of race science in the times of a public health crisis *Jon E.C. Tan*	70
six	It's just not cricket: (green) parks and recreation in COVID times *Kavyta Kay*	89
seven	Muslim funerals during the pandemic: socially distanced death, burial and bereavement experienced by British-Bangladeshis in London and Edinburgh *Farjana Islam*	109

eight	Racial justice and equalities law: progress, pandemic and potential *Robin Richardson*	129
nine	Out of breath: intersections of inequality in a time of global pandemic *Anon*	146
ten	An exploration of the label 'BAME' and other existing collective terminologies, and their effect on mental health and identity within a COVID-19 context *Ibiyemi Moshie-Moses*	157
eleven	COVID-19 in the UK: a colour-blind response *Jane Hinchcliffe*	176
twelve	Reviewing the impact of OFQUAL's assessment 'algorithm' on racial inequalities *Bruno Mallett*	187
thirteen	The impact of COVID-19 on Somali students' education in the UK: challenges and recommendations *Yusuf Sheikh Omar, Baar Hersi and Abdishakur Tarah*	199
Conclusion: Long COVID, long racism		216
Index		220

Notes on contributors

Sharon Anyiam is Lecturer in Health and Wellbeing in Society at De Montfort University and is completing her PhD in Sociology. Sharon has widespread experience in anti-racist community organising at grassroots level and, as a certifying doula, also has keen interest in fostering maternal health for minoritised ethnic and marginalised groups at a community level.

Baar Hersi is Assistant Principal in an inner London school, responsible for raising attainment, KS4 pastoral and DEI. She founded the British Somali Educators Association, a collective of Somali educators who are committed to establishing educational equity for Somali students and their communities.

Jane Hinchcliffe recently completed an MA in Race, Education and Decolonial Thought at Leeds Beckett University. She is a safeguarding professional specialising in work with both children and adults in the mental health sector and a self-employed parenting consultant, passionate about anti-racism, activism and working in solidarity with minoritised and underserved communities.

Tiffany R. Holloman is a project manager for Brad-ATTAIN and YCEDE in the Centre for Inclusion and Diversity at the University of Bradford. She is co-founder and co-director of Same Skies Think Tank, as well as a consulting lecturer at RADA in early modern history. Her sociological research examines race and education in the UK and US and her historical research investigates King James VI and I in Early Modern Britain. She is the author of several articles, chapters, as well as a co-editor of two books. Her activism stems from a desire to work with community members in the elevation of human development. She loves the arts, NES roms, travelling with her wife Toni, R&B, baseball, fishing and chess.

Farjana Islam is an urban practitioner and researcher with interests in exploring dynamics of social exclusion and inequalities that are experienced by vulnerable and disadvantaged communities in cities. Her doctoral research explored how the Olympic 2012 legacy-led regeneration was contributing to sociospatial and digital exclusions of minority communities in east London. Most recently, her research focuses on the challenges faced by Muslims in performing funerary rituals during the COVID-19 pandemic in the UK.

Kavyta Kay is Senior Lecturer in Race and Education at Leeds Beckett University. She received her PhD in Sociology from the University of Leeds and she was recently awarded a Senior Fellowship of the Higher Education Academy. Her teaching, writing and research interests lie in intersectional ways of thinking through race, gender and identity from multiple platforms namely academic, popular culture and social media. Her work, so far, has been on exploring discourses of decoloniality and South Asian identities in comedy, film, sport, education and, more recently, graphic novels.

Vini Lander is Professor of Race and Education and Director of the Centre for Race, Education and Decoloniality in the Carnegie School of Education. Vini's research focuses on race, ethnicity and education. She uses critical race theory as a theoretical framework to examine 'race' inequalities in education, specifically in teacher education.

Bruno Mallett is an emerging researcher in education studies. Since graduating from Leeds Beckett University in 2020, Bruno has progressed onto an MSc in Education at the University of Oxford. He continues to write on issues surrounding education from often philosophical and political perspectives.

Ibiyemi Moshie-Moses is a south Manchester-based artist filmmaker, womanist, student in decoloniality and waitress. Building on and developing from the introspection of her experimental film portfolio created during her time at Manchester School of Art, her interests in postgraduate academia currently lie in the relationship between ideology and identity: exploring 'race' and ideas around heteronormativity, class and categorical identity through an intersectional lens. Her most recent paper scrutinised and investigated the café as an institution that reproduces whiteness.

Yusuf Sheikh Omar is Research Associate at SOAS University of London, Global Advisor to Global Reconciliation, and Managing Director, ILAYSNABAD (Light of Peace): Dialogue & Development Initiative (IDDI). His research has focused on identity, and the social integration experiences of young diasporic Africans and Muslims into the West, as well as peace and nation building in the Horn of Africa.

Robin Richardson is a former director of the Runnymede Trust and the Insted Consultancy, and is the current manager of the latter's website at www.insted.co.uk. He is the author or editor of many publications on aspects of racism, Islamophobia and inequalities.

Javeria K. Shah is an interdisciplinary scholar and arts activist specialising in sociology, the arts, education and policy. She holds a range of academic and scholarly roles, including at the Royal Central School of Speech and Drama, University of London, and the University of Arts London. In 2018 she founded the Social Performance Network, a project organically grown out of her art, research, teaching and activism interactions. The Network collaborates with artists, activists, and academics to create such spaces and promotes an ethos of nuance to conversations relating to identity, including race.

LaTonia A. Siler-Holloman is a sociologist specialising in the Progressive Era Black professional of the US. A proud graduate of North Carolina Agricultural and Technical State University, Toni is a champion of historically black colleges and universities (HBCUs) and their importance in higher education. Through her company, Bside Professional Services, she advocates for the globalisation of HBCUs, expansion of international education, and support for postgraduate students. Her latest article, 'Education as a human right: the rise of the HBCUs', co-authored with her wife, Tiffany R. Holloman, is an exploration of the HBCU contribution to the political, economic and social uplift of the Black community.

Jon E.C. Tan is Senior Lecturer in Education at Leeds Beckett University. With a background in sociology, social policy, social welfare and politics, he has contributed to a wide range of research programmes centred on the examination of those inequalities that impact upon schools and their communities. Alongside his undergraduate and postgraduate teaching, he supervises doctoral studies and has been involved in professional learning and development in schools both in the UK and overseas. He is also a military historian and a musician.

Abdishakur Tarah is Lecturer and scholar activist in Education. He is a PhD candidate at the University of Buckingham. He worked as an education advisor in Leicester with a specific role in the prevention of school exclusion and parental involvement. He is a Fellow of the Higher Education Academy, and senior education consultant for the UK-based education consultancy Education Development and Support Services.

Tré Ventour-Griffiths is a practitioner-academic, as both a public historian of Black British history and a creative writer, with published work including journalism and (performance) poetry. He identifies as neurodivergent and disabled, and as a freelancer he has also delivered educational sessions on race, disability and Black British history to different sectors, including the arts, education and criminal justice. He has been interviewed by *The Guardian* and the BBC, and has written for big and small publications including *openDemocracy*, *NeuroClastic* and *Media Diversfied*.

Acknowledgements

The impetus for this edited collection came from the positive response to our initial call for papers for a special issue on COVID-19 and racism for the CRED (Centre for Race, Education and Decoloniality) working papers series. After some thoughtful conversations with CRED members, contributors and Bristol University Press, we decided to turn this into a book, and it is fitting that we owe thanks, first and foremost, to the authors who contributed to this collection. They all took time out of their busy schedules and challenging circumstances to help us realise our vision of compiling a record of how COVID-19 had impacted racialised communities, from a range of perspectives, and that would be accessible to a wide audience. The insights they generously shared is what will hopefully render this edited collection useful, and also intellectually stimulating.

Gratitude of a different but equally important nature goes to the Bristol University Press editorial staff who shepherded this project from the onset, and the reviewers whose thoughtful comments eased our way to completion.

Introduction: The long road ahead

On 31 December 2019, the world began to hear murmurs from the Chinese authorities and the World Health Organization (WHO) of the novel coronavirus, a mysterious new virus strain that had never been identified in humans. By 30 January 2020, WHO labelled SARS-Cov-2 (COVID-19) as a public health emergency of international concern. It did not take long (11 March 2020) for the widespread and rapidly evolving virus to be declared, a global pandemic.

If a pandemic is defined as 'a novel infection – new and previously unconfronted – that spreads globally and results in a high incidence of morbidity (sickness) and mortality (death)', deriving 'from *pan* – across, and *demos*, meaning people or population' (Doherty, 2013: 42), the new virus in this instance became confronted with an old one that has historical roots and continual contemporary manifestations – and that is the virus of racism. The antagonism, discrimination and prejudice directed against an individual of another race based on one's perceived racial superiority is not novel by any means. However, the histories of racism in the global North and South have never been more visible than in these pandemic times. Indeed, the impact of the latter on existing inequalities is wide-reaching, with reverberations felt worldwide. Even after three years since the arrival of COVID-19, many of the outcomes from these inequalities have been shown to be more exacerbated and devastating, particularly along the lines of race and ethnicity.

Global media discourses and scholarly debates have revealed over the course of 2020 onwards the role structural racism has played in perpetuating racial inequalities, and its impacts on Black and global majority groups has been laid bare. The COVID-19 pandemic has been a catalyst of many existing and intersectional issues globally, and it was with this in mind that the Centre for Race, Education and Decoloniality (CRED) at Leeds Beckett University initially issued a call for rapid response papers on the racial impacts of the coronavirus. More widely, we identified an emerging racist rhetoric of blaming and shaming Black, Asian and Minority ethnic groups, for instance in the conversations on vaccine hesitancy, higher COVID-19 incidence in Black communities, the labelling of the virus as the 'Chinese virus' and the 'Indian variant', to enumerate just a few examples.

In this spirit, this book is intended to make a meaningful contribution to Critical Race Studies by addressing the prejudices and explicit discrimination that emerge out of the collision of the two pandemics, namely COVID-19 and Racism, through a hybridised counter storytelling format. It seeks to examine the complexity of the collision of these pandemics, which become evident when examining the intersection between race, health, public policy and culture. The text takes an interdisciplinary approach to this by including submissions from students, researchers, teachers, educators and interested stakeholders, whose work connects to issues of activism, critical race and ethnic studies, community work, human geography, history and sociology. It is hoped this book will illuminate some aspects of how structural racism operates insidiously. We are thankful to both the authors for responding to our initial call and referees for their rigorous work. The contributions in this edited collection are an important intervention in speaking back to dominant discourses and the 13 chapters that make up this collection cover a range of facets that have been organised according to key themes to allow the reader to navigate the collection and weave connections as they go through the chapters.

To set the tone, we open with a spoken word piece by Javeria Shah, also available as an audio sample on the ebook version of this collection.

Through plotting a relationship to the Honours system via the COVID-19 pandemic and Black Lives Matter, the second chapter by Tré Griffiths makes a critical interrogation of the role of Honours in undermining pushes for equality, equity and justice. From his position as a Black-racialised man in the Black–white binary, he questions the motive of some people who accept Royal Honours. The Honours system is one that has been challenged on grounds of corruption (Bright, 2021). It brings a double threat: by legitimising white supremacy as ideology and Honours as an alleged corrupt system of merit. With both COVID-19 and Black Lives Matter, is it possible to become a life peer, and/or accept an empire medal, without accepting systems of violence?

The global majority has long been intimately aware of the health disparities in their communities. For the Black, Indigenous, Pacific Islander, and Latinx populations, distrust in the medical profession remains high due to centuries of traumatisation by white physicians and researchers in the US. As a result, these populations have been disproportionately represented in the morbidity and mortality rates, and their reticence to accept COVID-19 vaccinations posed a substantial risk to public health during the pandemic. The chapter by Tiffany R. Holloman and LaTonia A. Siler-Holloman focuses on Black reticence in the US. They charge that the 1910 Abraham Flexner report, grounded in the long history of Black inferiority and academic prestige hierarchy, was a major factor in the closure of the medical schools and hospitals of the historically Black colleges and universities, ending targeted services for people of colour. Using Critical Race Theory as a framework, they analyse the historical and contemporary consequences of the report, address its continuing role in the marginalisation of Black healthcare, and offer suggestions for medical social justice during the COVID-19 pandemic and beyond.

The fourth chapter, by Sharon Anyiam, takes an auto-ethnographic approach to understanding the impact of the pandemic and Black Lives Matter protests on Black millennial resistance. It analyses journal entries reflecting on the author's thoughts and feelings towards being a pregnant Black woman during a global pandemic that witnessed international Black Lives Matter protests, and discusses how Black millennials' experience of structural racism fostered a culture of resistance and activism during a global pandemic. This discussion builds on the scholarly discourse of Black resistance in the UK through the lens of a Black millennial mother.

Chapters 5, 6 and 7 provide a snapshot on Asian experiences in Britain during the COVID-19 pandemic. In 'It's alive! The resurrection of race science in the times of a public health crisis', Jon E.C. Tan explores how such institutional racism pervades public health responses to the health inequalities, highlighted in times of crisis. At its centre, it examines how the legacy of race science, a stark account being the high rates of anti-Asian hate crimes, casts long shadows across the ways in which patterns of vulnerability for BAME communities are acknowledged and then dismissed. Written from a British-born, mixed heritage perspective, the chapter engages with the issues of race, racism and the 2020 pandemic as a lived experience. Weaving together an analysis of the emerging evidence, reflective writing and storytelling, it suggests that the rivers of privilege and superiority run deep underneath the surface of public discourse. In doing so, it argues that a failure of public policy to directly address the disproportionality of vulnerability during the onset of this respiratory-debilitating virus has resulted in Black and global majority communities that could protest 'we can't breathe'.

The next chapter, by Kavyta Kay, shines a spotlight on the green space gap through the lens of park cricket, a sport widely played by South Asian communities across the UK. Over the course of the pandemic, the question of who gets to inhabit and access green spaces found resonance with historical and contemporary conversations on the status of Asians in cricket, both league and recreational, and this piece reflects on these spaces and conversations, where we see notions of privilege, imperialism, race and identity collide in particular ways.

The following chapter, by Farjana Islam, explores the challenges faced by Bangladeshi Muslims in relation to performing funeral and mourning rituals at community level, while adhering to the UK government's social distancing rules. Public Health England's analysis suggest that Bangladeshis, most of whom are Muslim, were disproportionately impacted by the COVID-19 infection. The findings discussed here include phone conversations with four Bangladeshi people who lost their friends or family during the pandemic and attended the burial and funeral rites of the deceased. The chapter narrates the funeral experiences and distresses, as well as the challenges and expectations, bestowed on the British-Bangladeshi community during the pandemic, in comparison to the ideal funeral rituals. The pandemic calls for innovative and expert-led planning interventions to prepare for similar situations in the future, with an enhanced collaboration between communities and the government.

The essential task when the pandemic is over will be not only to 'build back better', as the phrase goes, but also to build back fairer. If the new normal is not much fairer than previously, it will not, in fact, be better, and this is what Robin Richardson interrogates in Chapter 8, which embarks on an analysis of racial justice and equalities law. The Equality Act 2010 marked the culmination of 45 years of deliberation, argumentation, campaigning, advocacy, lobbying and legislating. It had the clear potential to reduce unlawful discrimination. Its most promising features in this respect included (1) a general duty it imposed on all public authorities not only to avoid adverse impacts on certain groups and communities, but also to promote greater equality of outcome among them; and (2) specific duties, the purpose of which was to support, focus and clarify the general duty. The two fields that had the greatest potential to make a significant impact on equality, namely health and education, were particularly dismissive and resistant over the course of the pandemic, and set about dismantling, or even totally abolishing, good practice that had been developed nationally and locally over the previous ten years. As a direct or indirect consequence of the government's indifference to race inequalities, disparities in education and in health massively increased. Bodies that might reasonably have been expected to raise their voices in protest, namely Her Majesty's Opposition and the Equality and Human Rights Commission, largely remained silent.

The next set of chapters focuses on intersections of inequality through a social lens of health. Never has the consonance of the phrase 'I can't breathe' struck such a profound chord and correlated to not only the symptoms of COVID-19 but also the suffocating nature of racism. This phrase was the world's condition for most of 2020, and one that leads to the question of who is able to breathe, as posed by two anonymous contributors in Chapter 9. The pandemic – which particularly affects the lungs – has exposed an intersection of pandemic and capitalism in which some bodies are affected more than others; research findings show that people of the global majority have been disproportionally impacted by coronavirus (University of Manchester, 2020). Simultaneously, the death of George Floyd and the pain of his final words, 'I can't breathe', have shown how the life-breath of some humans is more valued than that of others. This chapter draws on bell hooks' (1994: 130) notion of critical dialogue; a practice that involves 'individuals who occupy different locations ... mapping out terrains of commonality, connection and shared concern'. For hooks, this coming together in spirit of beloved community requires us to cross borders, thereby enriching each other's knowledge.

Ibiyemi Moshie-Moses explores the label 'BAME' and links between existing collective terminologies and their effects on identity and the collective mental health of communities other than white in the UK. It considers the existing literature on collective racial language, taking issue with current terms with attempts to methodically move towards a more Compassionate, Accurate, Linguistically sound and Contextually conscious (CALC) collective phrase for people who experience racism. Contextualising this topic in a COVID-19 social reality, the chapter notes the detrimental effect that the combination of a global pandemic that problematises 'BAME' people, and the ambiguity and confusion surrounding the term itself, have on individual and collective consciousness. It argues the need for a new collective term determined by the people the term describes; the result, however, is that an objective outcome cannot be achieved when dealing with identity and the subjective.

How does the concept of colour-blindness apply to the COVID-19 crisis? This pandemic has resulted in changes in all areas of society, employment, policing and, of course, healthcare. It has also served to highlight already present inequality in an alarming way. Health policy and practice is not an area that has somehow escaped structural racism. As a result, trust in the NHS and scientists has been damaged (Geddes, 2021) and for many, this can result in a reluctance to access healthcare. These harms have been caused by well-intentioned people conditioned by a society that privileges whiteness. Black pregnant women were eight times more likely to be admitted to hospital during the COVID-19 crisis than pregnant white women (NHS England, 2020). As the UK statistics have told us, COVID-19 disproportionately affects people of colour. The virus was initially touted by many in the press as the great leveller, which supposedly infected anyone at any time regardless of background or status. We quickly learned this was not the case. This virus operates in an unequal society, just as we all do. This chapter by Jane Hinchcliffe, highlights the way colour blind racism has worked in practice, using examples from public health and policing.

The final set of chapters turn our attention to the education system in Britain. Chapter 12 by Bruno Mallett looks at how English school closures, which lasted five months, led to an examination process in which individual grades were estimated through an algorithm and the metrics it was based on led to structural bias and racism. Although there remains a lack of available data, it is plausible to suggest that the algorithm significantly widened the 'attainment gap' in education. Though there is also an increasing plethora of research that focuses upon racial attainment gaps across the British system of education, both gaps will be referenced across this chapter to discuss the racial implications of the algorithm used by the Office of Qualifications and Examinations Regulation (OFQUAL), a non-ministerial government department that regulates qualifications, exams and tests in England. It highlights a need to abolish standardised assessments.

Continuing the focus on education, Yusuf Sheikh Omar et al's chapter is an examination of the impact of COVID-19 on Somali students' education in the UK. It describes the new set of challenges brought forward by the pandemic for a community that has already faced difficulties with regard to educational attainment in UK, due to a range of factors that the authors set out. They explore queries such as what were the key challenges encountering Somali-British students during lockdown?

References

Bright, S. (2021) 'How political corruption works in the UK', ByLine Times [online]. Available from: https://bylinetimes.com/2021/11/08/how-political-corruption-works-in-the-uk/

Doherty, P.C. (2013) *Pandemics: What Everyone Needs to Know*, Oxford: Oxford University Press.

Geddes, L. (2021) 'COVID vaccine: 72% of black people unlikely to have jab, UK survey finds', *The Guardian*, 16 January [online]. Available from: https://www.theguardian.com/world/2021/jan/16/COVID-vaccine-black-people-unlikely-COVID-jab-uk

hooks, b. (1994) *Teaching to Transgress: Education as the Practice of Freedom*, New York: Routledge.

NHS England (2020) 'NHS boosts support for pregnant black and minority ethnic women', *NHS England* [online]. Available from: https://www.england.nhs.uk/2020/06/nhs-boosts-support-for-pregnant-black-and-ethnic-minority-women/

University of Manchester (2020) 'Rapid evidence review: inequalities in relation to COVID-19 and their effects on London' [online]. Available from: https://data.london.gov.uk/dataset/rapid-evidence-review-inequalities-in-relation-to-COVID-19-and-their-effects-on-london

ONE

BLAME the BAME

Javeria Shah

I wrote this improvised piece in response to the UK government's delay in the release of their *Disparities in the risk and outcomes of COVID-19* report. Findings from the report identified disproportionately higher BAME mortality rates from COVID-19. The report concluded that 'COVID-19 is higher among people of BAME groups' (Public Health England, 2020: 39–40).

The delay of this report to the backdrop of a revival of Black Lives Matter (BLM) activism after the death of George Floyd compounded the issues surrounding everyday racisms. The delay of the report highlighted fears among UK officials of anti-racist uprising because of the glaring disparities in the report. Perhaps the biggest irony of all was that the very services that were supporting the public during this terrifying pandemic, services such as the NHS, were the very services mostly made up of Black and Brown employees. Public support was emerging not only within a racially hostile environment, but now a physically unsafe one. The irony continued when we were asked to nationally celebrate the NHS through neighbourhood cheers and applause – the imagery attached to the NHS was that of whiteness. The Black and Brown body, once more erased.

BLAME the BAME reflects my racial frustrations with us as a nation state, amid narratives of Brexit, COVID-19 and BLM – all compounded by the delay of this report which, when released, confirmed our fears as the melanated othered.

The piece speaks to the blame culture that often follows around the othered BAME, be it for the collapse of public services or the plight of the white working class. It speaks to the omissions of Black and Brown so intrinsic to our national-narratives, and the deliberateness of overlooking and dehumanising the othered BAME, which is an attitudinal hangover from our colonial past.

BLAME the BAME sheds light on the age-old trope of positioning the othered as sub-human, a threat, or a scapegoat – and invites the public to challenge such toxic narrativisations to really *see* and appreciate the people behind our services.

Blame the BAME

I teach your kids
I treat your sick
I clean your streets
I nurse your old
I am Black
I am Brown
Legacy, of your crown
After all I've done
You leave me to drown
You don't want me here
That much is so clear
All I get from you
Labels, Acronyms
Cluster me and mine
All in one safe swoop

Mute then Unmute x4
(Repeat) x16
Blame the BAME
Tame the BAME
Working your front line
We are dying
Stand Back
NHS must shine
Hide the Black
We are dying
Hide the brown
We are dying
Bring out eugenics
Silence your reviews
Dirty fascism
Hidden liberal truths
We are dying x2
Mute then Unmute x2
(Repeat) x8
Blame the BAME
Tame the BAME
We are dying
Hide the Black
We are dying
Hide the brown
Labels, Acronyms
Whitewash NHS
Bring out eugenics
Silence your reviews
(Repeat) x8
Blame the BAME
Tame the BAME

Reference

Public Health England (2020) 'Disparities in the risk and outcomes of COVID-19', PHE Publications [online]. Available from: https://www.gov.uk/government/publications/COVID-19-review-of-disparities-in-risks-and-outcomes

TWO

COVID-1984: wake MBE up when Black Lives Matter

Tré Ventour-Griffiths

Introduction

Coming from a creative writing background (mainly poetry), I have frequently used my art to discuss political and social problems. Seeing this chapter's title and the subheadings, many of you may think I also have a background in comedy! However, I promise I am not trying to be facetious; but I often use humour to make sense of serious issues. The title 'COVID-1984' not only encapsulates the seriousness of many preventable deaths (and ailments brought on by long COVID), but also the significance of intermittent lockdowns adjacent to the Black Lives Matter protests of 2020. Yet, this chapter's main topic is more insidious.

I argue that for some members of the public who were pivotal to the UK's COVID response then to be bestowed with Honours undermines governmental integrity. By 'Honours' I refer to the accolades given twice yearly by the Crown on recommendation from the Honours Committee, which is made of both government officials and private citizens (Cabinet Office, 2021). Honours is a carnival of mirrors, and I think it is problematic when people, who position themselves as anti-oppression, accept them.

For example, the acceptance of knighthoods by Professors Chris Whitty, Gregor Smith and Frank Atherton (Topping, 2021) from a country that, at the same time, has been underfunding the healthcare sector, seem duplicitous. Furthermore, allegations of political corruption have been noted within the Honours system itself (Bright, 2021).

With COVID-19 lockdowns widening inequalities, one must ask if it is appropriate for anybody to be buying into a system in the name of the British Empire – one of the biggest violators of human rights. These symbols of the empire matter, as 'even symbolic power is power because symbols give out messages to the world' (Renée Landell *qtd* in Al-Jazeera, 2022).

While I have named names in this chapter, I am not blaming these people. It is vital our analysis of Honours also considers the overarching system, because not only does this show how the public face of British Black Lives Matter is measured by its proximity to whiteness but, further, how organisations that had previously made anti-racism statements in 2020 in response to Black Lives Matter and the murder of George Floyd then dismissed those statements in their celebration of the Queen's Platinum Jubilee (Ventour, 2022). This cognitive dissonance pervades in the continued acceptance of Honours by many 'activists'.

I am boggled to see many people I have looked up to since childhood with those three letters hanging after their names like nooses – historians and creatives … and, um, campaigners and activists. Further concerning the pandemic, it was tough to watch COVID-19 doctors accept this form of state recognition (Duggan, 2020), as they were awarded by a government that gaslighted frontline workers for years, including healthcare staff and schoolteachers. Yet, I will concede that the pressure to conform in a capitalist society is overwhelming. As Nina Simone reportedly said in 1968:

> [I]t is difficult to retain your standards with the pressure of trying to make money, which always has its rules ... It's hard to walk the tightrope of doing what you think is your best and making money at it ... I have to constantly re-identify myself to myself, reactivate my own standards, my own convictions about what I'm doing and why.
> (Nina Simone *qtd* by Lexis, 2014)

Honours moving in parallel to the UK's COVID-19 response gives an indication of how power is transferred in this country, as we see when we consider the historic lineages of many of those inside those inner circles (further discussed in 'The Caucasian persuasion'). While in this chapter I focus on the lineages of Dominic Cummings and Dido Harding, it is worth acknowledging other ways colonialism, Honours and power intersect. For example, Conservative MP and Health Minister Edward Argar is a former lobbyist for Serco, the private company that was awarded numerous government contracts (Taylor, 2020). Serco's present CEO (as of July 2022), Rupert Soames, is the grandson of Sir Winston Churchill (Knight, 2015) and was made an Officer for the Order of the British Empire (OBE) in 2010 (London Gazette, 2009) – while his brother, Nicholas Soames, Conservative MP, was knighted in 2014 (London Gazette, 2014). On the one hand there is a discussion of Honours' links to senior COVID-19 jobs, while on the other there is a conversation that needs to be had about how those who accept Honours also hold some of the largest platforms on social justice issues, including anti-racism.

Through auto-ethnography, this chapter will look at my relationship to Honours via COVID-19 and Black Lives Matter. I think it is vital to juxtapose Britain's Honours system with not only Black Lives Matter but also the government's COVID-19 response. The former because it depicts how many of those positioned as 'the face of British anti-racism' in the summer of 2020 did so only within the realm of 'state respectability'. Their inclusion into the establishment gives white supremacy the greenlight, albeit symbolically. However, in relation to the allocation of senior COVID-19 jobs, we must think about the trajectory of the people into these jobs, some from families who have historically been part of Britain's gilded circles, considering the link between Honours and hereditary aristocracy since the 'fall' of empire. We cannot blame them for the actions of their antecedents (which in some cases involved services to colonialism), but what this does show is how history still impacts the present day, as discussed below in the section 'Crossing the (white) picket'.

It is important to note that, while my positionality will mainly be embedded in my experience of Black Lives Matter from the Black–white binary, it is not to invalidate other vital discussions – not only in terms of Britain's other racialised minorities and Honours, but also of white 'allyship', and its waxing and waning sentiments.

Crossing the (white) picket

The arrival of COVID-19 in the UK has illuminated which sector of people are vital to public wellbeing. Yet, the government's actions during the pandemic appear to have benefited hedge fund managers and estate agents (Dawkins, 2021) more than frontline workers – since assets, income and the ability to travel were markedly divided. From March 2020, we have witnessed the government's contempt for the public sector, specifically how the National Health Service (NHS) was sidelined during the government's COVID-19 response in favour of corporations (DDN, 2020a). Furthermore, the NHS, a tangible feature of British culture, is (as of July 2022) nearing its complete conversion into a US-style healthcare system, as the current Tory parliament prioritises maximising profits over the British public. Ironic.

However, this shredding of the NHS should not be a surprise, considering how senior roles in the government's COVID-19 response were allocated. For example, made a life peer in 2014, former-TalkTalk CEO Dido Harding was tasked with leading the test and trace system in May 2020; yet her grandfather, Sir John Harding, was given a hereditary peerage for his services to the British Empire in his suppression of anti-colonial uprisings (Time, 1956). He also worked, in the 1950s, with Sir Evelyn Baring, the grandfather-in-law of PM Boris Johnson's former aide Dominic Cummings (DDN, 2020b). Baring was Governor of Kenya when it was a British colony (see below, 'The Caucasian persuasion'). Both men were given state honours, thus projecting their descendants into the establishment's inner circles. While I do not blame Cummings or Harding for the actions of their forebears, what we must consider is how power in this country is transferred. As Ash Sakar says:

> [Britain has] ... a remarkably stable, consistent and resilient ruling class ... [and] ... the same monarchy (with a ... hiccup in the Civil War) for about 1200 years ... a hereditary aristocracy which still owns swathes of this country and has representation in ... the House of Lords. Because of that fact, I think we have ... this idea of our history being the ... reorganisation of chairs at the top of the dining club, rather than the heaves of history powered by working-class struggle and ... resistance. ... it's not just Henry VIII, ... Victoria, and ... Churchill – it's the Levellers, the Chartists, British Black Panthers, the Grunwick Strikes, the Miners' Strike ... That story does not get told very often because if you were to tell it too often, you would start asking uncomfortable questions about that ruling class which hasn't changed all that much since William the Conqueror. (DDN, 2021c)

Given how the monarchy is thought of in the UK, particularly in my experience, it has been difficult to challenge the monarchy without facing a backlash. I was told to stop 'inciting hatred' when I published an article in the Northamptonshire magazine, *The Nenequirer,* when I offered a contrasting perspective of the mainstream news concerning the Queen's Jubilee (Ventour, 2022). I was also told that 'if I didn't like Britain [meaning my critique of institutional accountability], then "leave"'. The backlash received felt reminiscent of the talks held by the Duke and Duchess of Sussex following their racism accusations against other members of the Royal Family (Lang, 2021), as if the history of the British Empire and its endorsement of the human trafficking of Black people could not possibly affect the actions and operation of Britain today (Sanghera, 2021: 12). Challenging racism is tough enough; challenging the Honours system may be harder still.

Amid discourses regarding COVID-19 and British wellbeing, the state continued to gaslight healthcare staff. At the same time, establishment broadcasters positioned 'respectability' as the face of anti-racism, as many Blacks were faced with a wellbeing crisis being both essential to Britain, yet Black. Does anti-racism need to be respectable? If anything, anti-racism on state terms is a red flag. As Chardine Taylor Stone wrote, 'Let's be honest, anyone … doing anything that is even vaguely seen as a threat to the status quo would not be nominated … in the first place' (@ChardineTaylor, 2021).

'Postcolonial banter'

Black inclusion on the Honours list seemingly reflects a reward system that celebrates Black achievement is terms of how well Black people assimilate into white systems of merit. Thus, Black claims to Britishness can have qualifiers attached. In my experience, I have seen this particularly within Black celebrations of Honours being synonymous with the 'euphoria' of being in proximity to (white) power. To be state-recognised is to be accredited as 'good citizens', very much entangled in the conceptualisation of 'good immigrants' (Shukla, 2016; Shukla and Suleyman, 2019). Many Black Brits chose assimilation into the system when they decided to accept entry onto the Honours list, just as many 'white allies' positioned themselves as pro-equality, while also taking empirical recognition.

For many of us who are British colonial descendants, these medals of colonial honourifics appear like a toxic friend in the closet – gaslit, manipulated, and lied to. As Guilaine Kinouani (2021: 56) writes:

> Although [respectability and assimilation] may provide temporary escape and possibly material gain and conditional access to structures of power, they produce white supremacy and such breed further shame and self-alienation. Self-contempt, disdain and scorn were not merely accidental by-products of colonialism – they were manufactured, deliberate colonial weapons to fortify whiteness and reduce resistance.

Guilaine's Kinouani's point holds weight. My interactions with many Black people, even of my parents' age group (born 1969–1974), show that they are traumatised by racism to the point they see proximity to whiteness as safety. Frantz Fanon first discussed internalised whiteness in *Black Skin, White Masks* (1952). In more contemporary times, 'This is Not a Humanising Poem' by Suhaiymah Manzoor-Khan (2019) also examines 'respectability' politics. For example, as a Black-racialised male, I am required to be 'overly polite' in white spaces to be seen as 'human'. While I do my utmost to be courteous always, that decision should not have qualifiers attached. Colloquial connotations of state honours do come with notions of civility, but the histories they are attached to are anything but. As I respect much of the work the recognised Black educators and practitioners delivered during the summer of 2020, it was challenging to be educated about inequalities, knowing full well these state privileges are something they will have to relinquish if we are to have an equitable society. After all, these medals are one of the continuing reminders of the British Empire.

Even more disconcerting, author-activist George Monbiot says, 'the highest award for British officials who work abroad is the Order of Saint Michael and Saint George' (DDN, 2020b: 0:00–0:08). The imagery presents a white angelic figure, standing on the head of the devil (the devil being a Black man). Monbiot goes on to liken it to 'a policeman kneeling on George Floyd's neck … the idea of standing or kneeling on the neck of a Black man is deeply embedded in these notions of dominance – of white people over Black people, the dominance of western nations over other countries' (0:26–0:44). In essence, these medallions (the Order included) reflect the social fabric Britain is built on, with whiteness as a master signifier (Seshadri-Crooks, 2000: 3–4).

One such example is Lord Kitchener, who anyone that went to school in the UK would have seen on the 'Your Country Needs You' 1914 wartime propaganda posters. Horatio Herbert Kitchener, 1st Earl Kitchener, was awarded numerous Honours in service to Britain, including 'The Most Distinguished Order of Saint Michael and Saint George' in 1900 (London Gazette, 1901). What we did not learn in school (or at least I did not) is of his 'colonial services' in South Africa. For example, near the climax of the Second Boer War, many Boer fighters facing defeat at the hands of the British adopted guerrilla tactics. In response, Kitchener actioned his scorched-earth policy, destroying civilian farms and homes to prevent the Boers from accessing food and supplies (Downes, 2007). When thinking about the sorts of people on the Honours list, even historically, is this a circle one would want to be part of? Furthermore, in the same conflict, Kitchener expanded (1st Earl) Lord Roberts' concentration camps (Pretorius, 2011). How can people who position themselves as anti-oppression take state honours in the name of a system that institutionalised white supremacy while also facilitating land grabs and genocide?

Moreover, while here it would be appropriate to talk about someone like Sir Winston Churchill (Kehinde Andrews, in GMB, 2018a; Afua Hirsch, in GMB, 2018b; Ross Greer, in GMB, 2019), Monbiot continues to name Sir Evelyn Baring, who as Governor of Kenya in the 1950s instituted 'a system of concentration camps which even his own attorney general compared to those run by the Nazis' (DDN, 2020b). Thus, when I think of Honours, it is wrapped in histories where colonisers and racists are awarded state recognition. The Order of Saints Michael and George, like other state honours, glorify colonial foot soldiers who have enabled or committed horrific acts of 'white terror' (hooks, 1992: 170). All while the contemporary perpetuation of the British Empire sits juxtaposed to the necessary challenge protesters brought to colonial statues in the summer of 2020 – especially when there are further instances; for example UK PM Boris Johnson tweeting that to pull down statues is 'to lie about our history' (@BorisJohnson, 2020). How can pulling down statues lie about history when Britain's highest system of merit is in the colonial white gaze?

Amid movements to decolonise curricula, educators have willingly taken Honours – one of the continuous symbols of colonialism in Britain. It is a reminder of 'respectability', where diverse 'overwhelmingly [means] the inclusion of people who look different' (Puwar, 2004: 1). Shona Hunter describes a white nation as a country whose identity, cultural practices, and economic relationships 'are enacted through the naturalisation of whiteness via processes of external (global "elsewhere") and internal (national "at home") colonisation of Black subjects' (2015: 44), while the Honours system concurrently reminds me how we are internally colonised. And since 'white' is often seen as unraced, 'If diversity becomes something that is added to organizations, like color, then it confirms the whiteness of what is already in place' (Ahmed, 2012: 33). Sara Ahmed's statements may apply to Honours where 'diversity' asserts the whiteness of the list already there.

In January 2022, the BBC reported: 'In total, 15.1% of recipients are from an ethnic minority background, which the government said made it "for the 4th time running, the most ethnically diverse honours list to date". In total, 47.9% of recipients are women' (Amos, 2022). So, the Royal Family is akin to many UK institutions, where diversity is marketing (Ahmed and Swan, 2006). By recognising more Black people, they try to change '*perceptions of whiteness rather than change the whiteness of* [the institution]. Changing perceptions of whiteness can be how an institution can reproduce whiteness, as that which exists but is no longer perceived' (Ahmed, 2012: 34). While there was a reported increase in racialised minorities being tapped for state recognition, the number of people rejecting Honours has doubled in the last ten years (Busby, 2020). However, in a 2014 YouGov survey, more than half (59%) of people polled thought the British Empire was a source of pride rather than shame (Dahlgreen, 2014). Post-Brexit, has anything changed? And through a 'diverse' list, the very existence of Honours celebrates how Britain still holds dominance over countries that they previously colonised. As comedian Trevor Noah states:

> The British did [colonisation] perfectly ... because now we're friends. We all speak the same languages; we even have games where we participate together. The Commonwealth Games ... There was nothing common about it. The wealth was in one place. Right, let's forget everything ... and let's play some games together.
> (John Bishop Show, 2015)

Trevor Noah's synopsis reminds me how comedians often (but not always ... yikes) have their finger on the political and social pulse. And while Black people are not physically shackled to the sugar economy anymore, the system of racial capitalism still exists. Nancy Leong (2013) writes that 'the process of racial capitalism relies upon and reinforces commodification of racial identity ... reducing it to another thing to be bought and sold'. In the UK, this appears as Black and other racialised minorities are disproportionately at the frontlines of the workforce whose labour can (un)arguably be seen as 'disposable'. Furthermore, at least as highlighted in conversations with colleagues, violent and exploitative systems of employment are often still 'othered' to the global South, the US, or Eastern Europe. Meanwhile, academic staff at British universities continue to strike in disputes over pay, pensions, and working conditions (Havergal, 2022). In short, the idea of this reality of violent employment conditions in this country is extradited from British realities – out of sight, out of mind. Yet, millions were killed under empire, and while Honours continues, there is no respect for the dead. Both soldiers and civilians. The late war veteran Harry Patch called war 'a calculated and a condoned slaughter of human beings' (DDN, 2021a), all while racial capitalism persists built on past colonial exploits. As Walter Rodney (1982: 88–89) wrote:

> [I]t can be affirmed without reservations that the white racism which came to pervade the world was an integral part of the capitalist mode of production ... Occasionally, it is mistakenly held that Europeans enslaved Africans for racist reasons. European planters and miners enslaved Africans for economic reasons, so that their labor power could be exploited ... Oppression of African people on purely racial grounds accompanied, strengthened, and became indistinguishable from oppression for economic reasons.

Rodney's and Leong's points respectively hold sway. From my own positionality, people that look just like me are being devoured by capitalism in a world where our bodies are tied to labour. While the frontlines of the NHS are disproportionately filled with Black and racialised minorities, one could argue the PPE scandal is also racist. However, there is an ideological

British exceptionalism to the idea that Britain could be corrupt – that is the debacle around PPE contracts, the Owen Paterson scandal and the PartyGate scandal at Number 10 (Helm et al, 2021; Transparency International, 2021; Walker, 2021). These incidents should have been treated as national crises, but were not. This 'exceptionalism' was most evident where I found colleagues more open to discussing corruption in the Indian government's COVID response (DDN, 2021e), but not in Britain's. Seemingly, I have found more people at ease discussing corruption in relation to the global South, particularly India and the African continent. British exceptionalism to corruption is stark, and often, but not always, reflective of the racist social fabric Britain is built on. Yet it is vital to remember this is not unprecedented.

The Caucasian persuasion

Operation Legacy was a British state-sanctioned disposal of colonial documents, to prevent them being inherited by now 'former colonies' (Cobain, 2016; Gilbert, 2016). It took place between the 1950s and 1970s, as countries began to fight for and assert their independence (Mustermann, 2014). However, today, I still find that the ambivalence to the Honours system is due to the state's systematic intentions to erase the British Empire from the national psyche. For example, I do not think Operation Legacy is in the minds of most educators. As Jeffrey Boakye tweeted, 'in a zoom call of over 100 experienced educators and sector professionals, little old me was the ONLY person who had heard of Operation Legacy' (@jeffreyboakye, 2021). Historic cover-ups of imperial crimes further underpin challenges to teaching empire as part of the national school curriculum. While we have a merit system that glorifies empire, simultaneously those who write the official history want Operation Legacy to remain an enigma.

At the same time, the way some have received Honours is dubious. As Byline Times editor Peter Jukes says, 'it is illegal to solicit honours/peerages in return for donations but ... you are highly likely to get [one] – in fact 55% of those who donated more than £1.5m get an honour or a peerage' (DDN, 2021b). Furthermore, in 2016, former PM David Cameron was challenged when he was found to have awarded Tory donors Honours, and former PM Theresa May faced calls 'to block honours for No 10 "cronies" after a leaked list revealed David Cameron ... requested knighthoods for party donors, pro-EU campaigners and political aides' (Mason, 2016).

Dating back to the mid-noughties, former Labour PM Tony Blair was also criticised when a 'sleaze watchdog ... blocked [his] list of 28 life peerages pending a "cash for favours" probe' (Lidstone, 2005). While in 2021, over one million people signed a petition to revoke his knighthood after he was tapped for recognition to be made a Knight of the Garter (Atkinson and Forrest, 2022). What this shows is the Honours system is not only part of the British Empire's legacy, but alive to contemporary political and economic dynamics across the political spectrum.

While the Honours system can be seen to be corrupt, there are many that do receive them for wholesome contributions; for example, those who receive them for community work. Sports journalist Jeff Stelling believes that Honours should go to people who go above and beyond for their community and should not go 'to someone for doing their job well and being paid for it ... the rich and famous ... sportsmen or women for simply winning things ... political cronies' (Sky Sports Retro, 2022). However, are colonial honourifics to the British Empire fitting merits of achievement in a society (or at least some parts of society) that claims to be modern and forward-thinking? Whether we are talking about community heroes or rich celebrities, those empire medals should leave a sour taste in anyone's mouth.

Yet, concurrently, following the murder of George Floyd, with reinterest in anti-racism (performative or otherwise), I was concerned to see people queueing up for their gong while public consultations were being conducted into colonial statues and streets named after racists and colonisers. What is more, I was concerned to see those who had taken Honours for combatting the varied institutional violence manufactured and/or upheld by the state, including services to eradicating poverty and racism, and further to charity and combatting other inequalities, after many across the country had marched that summer in solidarity with Black Lives Matter. The fact charity exists is really an indicator of either the disproportionate distribution of wealth in this country, and/or a failure of government. Honours for charitable services is as much a contradiction as nods for tackling racism, poverty and other forms of violence.

Particularly following *Small Axe* (2020), *Statue Wars: One Summer in Bristol* (2020) and *Uprising* (2021), I was challenged to think how anybody could consciously take these medallions knowing the discourses these programmes are intertwined with – the legacies of enslavement and colonialism. Also, after watching Charlene White's *Empire's Child* (2021), these split feelings became greater still, as much of the popular media narratives made about racism, including documentaries, are made by people who have accepted inclusion onto the Honours list. All the while the *Sewell Report* further ridiculously told us that there is no evidence of institutional racism (White and Coweburn, 2021). And at the same time, 2021 and 2022 boasted diversity in the Honours nominations, interlocking with how the monarchy increased the numbers of nominated racialised minorities as a smokescreen for the accusations of racism that followed Meghan and Harry's interview with American talk show host Oprah Winfrey.

During the pandemic, I found many people reliant on the arts to live. Locked down, the work of creatives across genres touched many (while the government at the same time gutted the arts and culture industry). However, watching recognised Black creatives being commissioned by establishment broadcasters, it was not difficult to see how 'respectability' plays a role in who gets entrusted to be the mouthpieces of Black Britain in popular media. Unbeknown to me then, this was celebrity activism (Coley, 2020), where I witnessed many of those educating us on racism also had those three letters after their names, hanging like nooses. However, this is not exclusively a Black problem; it is a people problem. Particularly amid the euphoria of Black Lives Matter, these protest chants took place while simultaneously recognising that few want to let go of their privileges. This shows the relationship between cognitive dissonance, Honours, and inclusion into whiteness. As Tao Leigh Goffe tweeted 'so often the price of inclusion is allowing yourself to be used as a pawn against your own people or those you should be in solidarity with' (@taoleighgoffe, 2021). Ultimately, this further centres the relationship between diversity and institutional whiteness (Ahmed, 2012), as those actually challenging the powerful are unlikely to be recognised (@ChardineTaylor, 2021). Why are some Black people so eager to be in proximity to power, when the long tables in executive boardrooms have often acted against our interest? Perhaps it would be more useful to find solidarity on the street level. As Ash Sakar says:

> The problem with liberal identity politics is that it puts recognition from the state above self-organisation and above collective struggle and above solidarity. So, if we want those ingredients to mean anything we've got to divest ourselves of the desire to be recognised by those at the top and start recognising each other.
>
> (DDN, 2021c)

(Black) British Empire? Dash weh!

Although some who live in my locality, Northamptonshire, have taken Honours, this is not always a reflection on values, as their work has been instrumental to different causes. However, the notion of more Black faces in high places as an antidote for a racist society is flawed, when we have seen that Black people in leadership can also act like their managers. Yet, despite the noble intentions of many (not just Black) members of the Honours list, the integrity of that system is compromised due its colonial roots and further criticisms of corruption.

In 2003, Benjamin Zephaniah declined an OBE due to its colonial links (Zephaniah, 2003). Activist Gina Martin rejected an OBE in 2020 saying 'It would be deeply hypocritical … to accept this honour while continuing to be vocal in my commitment to anti-racism' (Busby, 2020). However, they are the exception and, with so many Black and non-Black people also measuring their worth in proximity to imperialist white supremacist cisnormative heteropatriarchal power structures, I must ask whether they believe pushes for equality are less valuable than state recognition? While it is too easy to stigmatise individuals, it would be more useful to focus on how Britain has a corrupt imperialist system of recognising many legitimate achievements. Meanwhile, members of the public, including activists, continue to accept British Empire medals, undermining the integrity of all pushes for social justice and genuine lasting change.

The Honours system is a reminder of an elongated colonial history and parallel histories of corruption. If nominees do not boycott, can we even say Black lives matter? Change has rarely come from the top; it has more often been bottom-up by public demand. Aside from anti-colonial arguments, there is an anti-corruption argument that we may not have considered, but ought to – especially in a pandemic mired by scandal. Change is possible with a demand, and it is possible to give Honours back, as actor Michael Sheen did in 2017 (Rawlinson, 2020).

Conclusion

In conclusion, since March 2020 we have seen the double threat of Honours via not only its histories in empire, but further, its integrity embroiled by corruption. In recent times, medical doctors have accepted Honours from the same British government that refused to pay NHS workers fairly and is hellbent on dismantling the NHS itself – this is one example of how ordinary people have investment. And this comes while some nurses are being forced to use foodbanks. In education, it is unsettling to see how some educators pontificate about equality and justice while taking empire medals. As one Twitterer writes 'I truly don't understand the cognitive dissonance it takes to accept an OBE & simultaneously talk about anti-oppression' (@TweetsBilal). At every stage of education, how can we talk about decolonisation or anti-racism while there are still people (of all backgrounds) looking for inclusion into the empire project? This is colonialism's long reach in Operation Legacy 2.0. As Churchill said at the dawn of the Battle of Britain, 'If the Empire lasts a thousand years men will say, this was their finest hour' (War Illustrated, 1940: 686–687).

This chapter has sought to discuss my view of the walking contradictions of the many who talk about equality while also accepting British Empire medals. Yet, while Honours are a reminder of empire, like-violence continues today, including the settler colonialism happening in the Israelis occupation of Palestine (DDN, 2021f). And to live in a UK where many talk of anti-oppression while Honours persist, is to disrespect the dead. And, what is more, to dishonour the living.

Our ancestors are spinning in their graves.

References

@BorisJohnson (2020) 'They had different perspectives, different understandings of right and wrong. But those statues teach us about our past, with all its faults ...', *Twitter*, 12 June.

@ChardineTaylor (2021) 'Let's be honest, anyone whose doing anything that is even vaguely seen as a threat to the status quo would not be nominated for these "honours" ...', *Twitter*, 12 June.

@jeffreyboakye (2021) '… in a zoom call of over 100 experienced educators and sector professional, little old me was the only person who had heard of Operation Legacy …', *Twitter*, 14 March.

@taoleighgoffe (2021) 'So often the price of inclusion is allowing yourself to be used as a pawn against your own people or those you should be in solidarity with', *Twitter*, 1 October.

@TweetsbyBilal (2020) 'I truly don't understand the cognitive dissonance it takes to accept an OBE & simultaneously talk about anti-oppression', *Twitter*, 5 June.

Ahmed, S. (2012) *On Being Included*, London: Duke.

Ahmed, S. and Swan, E. (2006) 'Doing diversity', *Policy Futures in Education*, 4(2): 96–100.

Al-Jazeera English (2022) 'The UK is celebrating 70 years of Queen Elizabeth the Second | Inside Story', YouTube [online]. Available from: https://www.youtube.com/watch?v=cMCY6I7HOsc

Amos, O. (2022) 'New Year Honours: Whitty, Van-Tam and Blair knighted, Lumley and Redgrave made dames', *BBC News* [online]. Available from: https://www.bbc.co.uk/news/uk-59809682

Atkinson, E. and Forrest, A. (2022) 'Tony Blair: 1 million petition to "rescind" knighthood from former PM', *Independent* [online]. Available from: https://www.independent.co.uk/news/uk/tony-blair-petition-knighthood-b1988822.html

Bright, S. (2021) 'How political corruption works in the UK', ByLine Times [online]. Available from: https://bylinetimes.com/2021/11/08/how-political-corruption-works-in-the-uk/

Busby, M. (2020) 'Number of people rejecting Queen's honours doubles in past decade', *The Guardian* [online]. Available from: https://www.theguardian.com/politics/2020/dec/01/number-of-people-rejecting-queens-honours-doubles-in-past-decade

Cabinet Office (2021) 'Honours committees', Gov.uk [online]. Available from: https://www.gov.uk/guidance/honours-committees

Cobain, I. (2016) *The History Thieves*, London: Granta.

Coley, J. (2020) '"I take responsibility" and the limits of celebrity activism', New Yorker [online]. Available from: https://www.newyorker.com/culture/cultural-comment/i-take-responsibility-and-the-limits-of-celebrity-activism

Dahlgreen, W. (2014) 'The British Empire is "something to be proud of"', YouGov [online]. Available from: https://yougov.co.uk/topics/politics/articles-reports/2014/07/26/britain-proud-its-empire

Dawkins, D. (2021) 'UK billionaires are collectively $61 billion richer than a year ago', Forbes [online]. Available from: https://www.forbes.com/sites/daviddawkins/2021/04/07/uk-billionaires-are-collectively-61-billion-richer-than-a-year-ago/?sh=11f5012e2c54

Double Down News [DDN] (2020a) 'George Monbiot exposes COVID-19 corruption at the heart of government', YouTube [online]. Available from: https://www.youtube.com/watch?v=M4NNb0fmKR4

—— (2020b) 'Everything you know about the British Empire is a lie', YouTube [online]. Available from: https://www.youtube.com/watch?v=fSLDGuBPxJo

—— (2021a) 'Former soldier DESTROYS what Remembrance Day has become', YouTube [online]. Available from: https://www.youtube.com/watch?v=SrNpxcoj4f8

—— (2021b) 'There's a sickness at the heart of British democracy & it's called oligarchy', YouTube [online]. Available from: https://www.youtube.com/watch?v=_3PvOvLQrjA

—— (2021c) 'This is England: Ash Sarkar's alternative race report', YouTube [online]. Available from: https://www.youtube.com/watch?v=NFNiTcFbNu0

—— (2021d) 'How community organising could change the game for the British left', YouTube [online]. Available from: https://www.doubledown.news/watch/2021/30/march/why-community-organising-could-change-the-game-for-the-british-left

—— (2021e) 'Who is Boris Johnson's REAL boss?', YouTube [online]. Available from: https://www.youtube.com/watch?v=tqOa74dYO1g

—— (2021f) 'ISRAEL EXPOSED: colonialism, war crimes & the global far right', YouTube [online]. Available from: https://www.youtube.com/watch?v=OPPAfhamioc

Department of Health and Social Care (2020) 'New chair of COVID-19 "test and trace" programme appointed', Gov.uk [online]. Available from: https://www.gov.uk/government/news/new-chair-of-coronavirus-test-and-trace-programme-appointed

Downes, A.B. (2007) 'Draining the sea by filling the graves: investigating the effectiveness of indiscriminate violence as a counterinsurgency strategy', *Civil Wars*, 9(4): 420–444.

Duggan, J. (2020) 'Queen's Birthday Honours List 2020: every recipient of an award from Her Majesty from Northamptonshire', Northampton Chronicle [online]. Available from: https://www.northamptonchron.co.uk/news/people/queens-birthday-honours-list-2020-every-recipient-of-an-award-from-her-majesty-from-northamptonshire-2999246

Fanon, F. (1952) *Black Skin, White Masks*, London: Pluto Press.

Gilbert, R. (2016) 'Erasing empire', Jacobin [online]. Available from: https://jacobin.com/2016/11/british-empire-kenya-oman-ireland-state-secrecy

Good Morning Britain [GMB] (2018a) 'Is It Offensive to Quote Churchill?', YouTube [online]. Available from: https://www.youtube.com/watch?v=eoP4KuKOIuM

—— (2018b) 'Should we be ashamed of Winston Churchill?', YouTube [online]. Available from: https://www.youtube.com/watch?v=XhXoAkW9i88

—— (2019) 'Piers gets into a fiery debate over Scottish MP's Churchill comments', YouTube [online]. Available from: https://www.youtube.com/watch?v=Iy8Bt_V971o

Havergal, C. (2022) 'Ten more universities face strikes after UCU reballots', Times Higher Education [online]. Available from: https://www.timeshighereducation.com/news/ten-more-universities-face-strikes-after-ucu-reballots

Helm, T. et al (2021) 'Return of the sleazy party: the Conservatives and the Owen Paterson affair', *The Guardian* [online]. Available from: https://www.theguardian.com/politics/2021/nov/07/return-of-the-sleazy-party-the-conservatives-and-the-owen-paterson-affair

hooks, b. (1992) *Black Looks: Race and Representation*, Boston: South End Press.

Hunter, S. (2015) 'Being called to 'By the Rivers of Birminam': the relational choreography of white looking', *Critical Arts*, 29(1): 43–57.

John Bishop Show, The (2015) Episode 1. [Box of Broadcasts], 30 May, London. BBC One.

Kinouani, G. (2021) *Living While Black*, London: Penguin.

Knight, S. (2015) 'Can Winston Churchill's grandson save Serco? And is it worth saving?', *The Guardian* [online]. Available from: https://www.theguardian.com/business/2015/jul/02/serco-rupert-soames-outsourcing-privatisation

Lang, C. (2021) 'The core message of Meghan and Harry's Oprah interview: racism drove us from the Royal Family', TIME [online]. Available from: https://time.com/5944613/meghan-markle-oprah-racism/

Leong, N. (2013) 'Racial capitalism', *Harvard Law*, 126(8): 2153–2226.

Lexis (2014) 'The real Nina Simone', 1968 interview in *Down Beat Magazine*, *Music is My Sanctuary* [online]. Available from: https://www.musicismysanctuary.com/real-nina-simone-1968-interview-beat-magazine

Lidstone, J. (2005) 'The New Year Honours List is a corrupt farce', *Independent* [online]. Available from: https://www.independent.co.uk/voices/commentators/john-lidstone-the-new-year-honours-list-is-a-corrupt-farce-520923.html

London Gazette, The (1901) Issue 27306 [online]. Available from: https://www.thegazette.co.uk/London/issue/27306/page/2701

—— (2009) Supplement 59282. [online]. Available from: https://www.thegazette.co.uk/London/issue/59282/supplement/1

—— (2014) Supplement 60895 [online]. Available from: https://www.thegazette.co.uk/London/issue/60895/supplement/b1

Manzoor-Khan, S. (2019) *Postcolonial Banter*, Birmingham: Verve.

Mason, R. (2016) 'Cameron's "cronies" honours list leads to calls for overhaul of system', *The Guardian* [online]. Available from: https://www.theguardian.com/politics/2016/jul/31/remain-campaign-leaders-tory-donors-honours-david-cameron

Mustermann, E. (2014) 'Operation Legacy: how Britain destroyed thousands of colonial files', War History [online]. Available from: https://www.warhistoryonline.com/war-articles/operation-legacy-britain-destroyed-thousands-colonial-files.html?chrome=1

Pretorius, F. (2011) 'The Boer Wars', BBC History [online]. Available from: https://www.bbc.co.uk/history/british/victorians/boer_wars_01.shtml

Puwar, N. (2004) *Space Invaders*, London: Bloomsbury.

Rawlinson, K. (2020) 'Michael Sheen returned OBE to air views on royal family', *The Guardian* [online]. Available from: https://www.theguardian.com/culture/2020/dec/29/michael-sheen-gave-back-obe-to-air-views-on-royal-family

Rodney, W. (1982) *How Europe Underdeveloped Africa*, Washington, DC: Howard.

Sanghera, S. (2021) *Empireland*, London: Penguin.

Seshadri-Crooks, K. (2000) *Desiring Whiteness*, London: Routledge.

Shukla, N. (2016) *The Good Immigrant*, London: Unbound.

Shukla, N. and Suleyman, C. (2019) *The Good Immigrant USA*, London: Unbound.

Sky Sports Retro (2022) 'Jeff Stelling's New Year Honours rant', YouTube [online]. Available from: https://www.youtube.com/watch?v=Kz5qOqNoXPE

Taylor, D. (2020) 'Serco wins COVID-19 test-and-trace contract despite £1m fine', *The Guardian* [online]. Available from: https://www.theguardian.com/world/2020/jun/06/serco-wins-covid-19-test-and-trace-contract-despite-1m-fine

Time Magazine (1956) 'CYPRUS: Deepening Tragedy', *Time* [online]. Available from: https://tinyurl.com/w226vpmm

Topping, A. (2021) 'New year honours feature Covid experts with Chris Whitty knighted', *The Guardian* [online]. Available from: https://www.theguardian.com/uk-news/2021/dec/31/chris-whitty-knighted-as-covid-experts-feted-in-new-year-honours-list

Transparency International (2021) 'Track and Trace: identifying corruption risks in UK public procurement for the COVID-19 pandemic', *Transparency.org.uk* [online]. Available from: https://tinyurl.com/2eckfes8

Tuck, E. and Yang, W.Y (2012) 'Decolonization is not a metaphor', *Decolonization: Indigeneity, Education & Society*, 1(1): 1–40.

Ventour, T. (2022) 'God save the people: when will Black lives matter?', NQ [online]. Available from:https://nenequirer.com/2022/06/09/tre-ventour-asks-if-you-can-support-black-lives-matter-and-the-monarchy-in-thought-provoking-essay/

Walker, P. (2021) 'Chatting over cheese and wine: anatomy of Downing Street lockdown gathering', *The Guardian* [online]. Available from: https://www.theguardian.com/politics/2021/dec/19/chatting-over-cheese-and-wine-anatomy-downing-street-lockdown-gathering-picture

War Illustrated, The (1940) 'If the Empire lasts a thousand years', *War Illustrated* [online], pp 686–687

White, N. and Cowburn, A. (2021) ' "Institutional racism doesn't exist," government's race commission suggests in landmark report', *Independent* [online]. Available from: https://www.independent.co.uk/news/uk/politics/race-commission-report-institutional-racism-b1824605.html

Zephaniah, B. (2003) 'Me? I thought, OBE me? Up yours, I thought', *The Guardian* [online]. Available from: https://www.theguardian.com/books/2003/nov/27/poetry.monarchy

THREE

Black vaccination reticence: HBCUs, the Flexner Report and COVID-19

LaTonia A. Siler-Holloman and Tiffany R. Holloman

Introduction

Before COVID-19 was declared a pandemic by the World Health Organization in March 2020, Black and Brown people, who comprise the global majority,[1] experienced health disparities in their communities. The saying 'when white folks catch a cold, Black folks get pneumonia' is an apt gibe about the healthcare system efficacy in the US. Black communities absorbed the greatest blows from the pandemic due to their existing health challenges, disproportionate representation in the essential industries, pandemic communication gaps, and socioeconomic disparities (Tai et al, 2021: 705–706).

A Pew Research study found that, compared with Hispanic, white and Asian Americans, only 42 per cent of Blacks planned to get the COVID-19 vaccine (Funk and Tyson, 2020). Though reasons varied, Black people generally blamed the long history of medical malfeasance by government representatives, medical professionals and pharmaceutical executives for their mistrust in the COVID-19 vaccine; being more concerned about patterns of medical abuse and COVID-19 vaccine misinformation than actual viral infection.

Blacks, as well as other marginalised groups, are often positioned between the tension of actively building healthy lives and negotiating untrustworthy healthcare systems. We charge that their challenges are partially the result of an evaluation of medical schools by Abraham Flexner in 1910. Grounded in the 'Black inferiority' and 'academic prestige hierarchy' myths, Flexner's analysis of schools were warped by his ideologies on race and racism.

We chose the controversial[2] Critical Race Theory (CRT) to revisit the Progressive Era context of the 1910 Flexner report; the racialised closure of Historically Black College and University (HBCU) medical schools; and the continuing impacts of the closures on Black medical professionalism and Black healthcare. As race was integral in shaping the policies Flexner and various prominent white men endorsed regarding Black higher education, it is fitting that CRT is used to highlight truths behind this so-called period of 'progress'.

Using the Critical Race lens

Critical Race scholars observed patterns of political restraint and rights retraction after the Civil Rights Movement. They noticed the roles legal academics and practitioners played in the creation of statutes that reproduced political, economic and social oppression (Freeman, 1995). From their readings and analysis of the legal language, the founders of CRT articulated specific tenets to delineate the phenomenon they observed. The centrality of racism, whiteness as property, convergence of interest, critique of liberalism, perspectives of intersectionality, voices of Black and Brown people, and power of social justice would guide the interrogation of racial strategies used to subjugate, while highlighting the Black community tools used to thwart discriminatory policies.

For this chapter, we delve into the ways racism is embedded into US higher education and healthcare systems, showing how dominant narratives of Black inferiority and academic prestige hierarchy served to exclude Black representation in the medical industry. Despite the Progressive Era liberal policies implemented to uplift the fledging free Black community, we also highlight how racism becomes evident in the 'outcome of processes and relations irrespective of intent' (Rollock and Gillborn, 2011: 3).

The myths

Black inferiority

The common denominator of both the healthcare and educational systems of the US is the embeddedness of the Black inferiority myth. Black inferiority is the belief that people of African descent are intellectually, emotionally, physiologically and spiritually subordinate to the white people who inhabit the top of the racial hierarchy.

The lineage of the Black inferiority ideology in the US extends from the works of Plato and Aristotle. Plato, the founder of the Academy, commented on the honourable act of procreation as a civic duty and the limitation of 'inferior' citizens' rights to marriage and childbirth to inhibit degeneration of the population (Plato, n.d.; Galton, 1998; Siler-Holloman, 2020). De facto and de jure familial policies, such as abortion and infanticide, advocated by the philosophers and their fellow society members, secured control of the political, economic and social hierarchy for those in the upper echelons of the state. While early eugenic thought emphasised a hierarchy of physiological health, strength and ability, 'racial differences have perhaps nowhere escaped observation and comment' (Reuter, 1945: 453).

From the Middle Ages to the Enlightenment, Europeans judged others by their cultural practices and class status. Although debatable, European attitudes towards Blacks changed from xenophobia into a racialised ideology due to three significant factors: the indoctrination of Spanish *limpieza de sangre* or blood purity ideology; the creation of colonial societies in the 'New Worlds'; as well as, the European development of the transatlantic slave trade (Jordan, 1968; Barth, 2010; Burk, 2010). Academics from the Enlightenment shifted from theological and cultural explanations for human differences to the biological. Their conclusions from Linnaeus' (1758) work on the classification of species eventually expanded into the development of racial theoretical policies of 'differential treatment' of various groups, also known as pseudo-biological sciences (Reuter, 1945).

In the nineteenth century, biological theory became rife with issues, including questionable methodologies, logical fallacies and unethical practices, when scientists included subjective human traits in their research (Allen, 1983). According to the British scientist Francis Galton, eugenics is 'the science which deals with all influences that improve the inborn qualities of a race', so that 'the useful classes' 'should be better fitted to fulfil [their] vast imperial opportunities' (Galton, 1904: 1, 3). Recalling the ancient Greek philosophical beliefs, he posited, based on his 1869 work studying the pedigrees of prominent British families, that the best human qualities were found within the upper class of the Caucasian race (Allen, 1983; Norrgard, 2008). Despite the flaws, in the US, biologist Charles C. Davenport expanded upon Galton's work, establishing in 1910 the Eugenic Record Office (ERO), a breeding ground for the study, collaboration and public education of eugenics. His research institute was funded by philanthropists Mary Williamson Harriman, who inherited an amount valued in 2021 at $2 trillion, and Andrew Carnegie, through the Carnegie Institution of Washington, an organisation that supported scientific ventures (Allen, 1986: 235–236).

In his studies of the American Eugenics Movement, Garland E. Allen explained that the human hierarchies drawn by Galton and Davenport are value-judgment rankings that originated outside of biology. Allen specified that 'the notion of "value" … is crucial, for it is the basis on which the hierarchy is constructed in the first place, and is thus inherent in its use value' (Allen, 1983: 106). The value form (wealth or prestige) may vary for different hierarchies; however, the central principle holds – objects or groups of the higher levels have greater value than the lower (Allen, 1983). Allen argued that eugenic researchers created the socially-constructed rank order hierarchy of human attributes and presented them 'in the guise of the more scientific-appearing aggregational hierarchy', noting the chronic influence on 'biological thinking' (Allen, 1983: 107). Black people were listed at the lowest level of this hierarchy.

The placement and influence of proponents of eugenics allowed for local, state and federal government to enact laws protecting 'desirable' members of society. In 1927, in *Buck v Bell*, the US Supreme Court upheld involuntary sterilisation policies, and by 1939 30 states had codified compulsory sterilisations of the 'unfit' into law (Reilly, 2015: 355). Race-based immigration quotas and minimum wage requirements were thought to safeguard 'deserving workers from the competition of the unfit', 'who even after having received special training, remain incapable of adequate self-support' (Seager, 1913: 9–10; Leonard, 2005: 213, 219).

Difference within societies has been a constant. Yet, as exhibited by the *limpieza de sangre* or blood purity ideology and laws of fifteenth-century Spain, during times of national instability from immigration, civil war, diverse religious presences and resource depletion, native stakeholders align to preserve traditions, protect identity and eliminate financial competition from the 'others' (Burk, 2010; Siler-Holloman, 2020). Black inferiority is an example of what CRT scholars identify as 'master narratives' – ideologies that present the experience of the dominant group as normative and universal created to support these goals. In the US, the continuing industrial revolution, Civil War recovery, slave emancipation, and dire national debts owed to European investors contributed to the instability in the US (Jaynes, 1986: 11) . The 'scientific' validation of Black inferiority through eugenics provided the mechanism to retain political, economic, and social control in the Progressive Era.

Academic prestige hierarchy

Academic prestige hierarchy (APH) is another narrative that became prominent in the Progressive Era. APH is an assumption and belief that certain highly ranked institutions are the best in the educational system. The illusionary ranking system is controlled by a network of elite group members that only allow access to select members of their league. As exclusivity increases, so does the academic prestige (Holloman, 2019).

The hierarchy was problematic on several levels. The elite group members alone determined the ranking of the institutions, inevitably placing their schools of interest at the top. The students who were typically admitted to the top-ranked schools were elite group members. The networks developed to support the elite students were closed to outsiders. Many of their graduates did not altruistically work toward the betterment of society; rather, they strove to preserve their elite status and financial security (Holloman, 2019). Randall Collins described the categorisation and consolidation of higher education as a 'nativist counterattack'; a way for Anglo-Protestant men to control the professional class and dominate opportunities (Collins, 2019).

The CRT tenet of 'whiteness as property' assigns meaning to the APH. Whiteness as property refers to the conscious or unconscious ways in which white privilege – the dominant control of resources and ideas – is created and reproduced throughout society (Harris, 1993; Rollock and Gillborn, 2011). The emergence of land-grant universities across the US for the public and the founding of HBCUs promised to produce generations of professionals, including Blacks, who would compete for employment positions previously held by the upper class. As will be exhibited in the following sections, the dominant class members constructed a ranking hierarchy of universities to maintain superior status within the Academy.

The realities
Land-grant colleges and universities

The Morrill Acts of 1862 and 1890 represented the national desire for advancement in both education and industry. The Acts designated federal government provisions of land and funds to each state for the establishment of public colleges and universities for the 'common' man (Siler-Holloman, 2020). Although the colleges and universities have greatly contributed to technological innovations, critical scholars renamed the institutions 'land-grab universities' for the problematic history of government fraud and theft of Native American property for the scheme (Lee and Ahtone, 2020).

Out of nearly 50 predominately white land-grant colleges and universities, only eight of those institutions allowed Black people to graduate (Holloman, 2019: 83). While the aim of the second Morrill Act was the higher education of white citizens, the legislators specified federal funds to states for the advanced education of the Black community, institutions now known as HBCUs. 'If race was an admissions factor at the existing state university', then officials were to provide separate institutions for Black students (Association of Public and Land-Grant Universities, 2019). Given the choice, state representatives initially opened 19 HBCUs with the funding. Fourteen HBCU medical schools were established between 1865 and 1923 (Savitt, 1987).

By 1917, researchers found that the curriculum of the land-grant universities across the nation included eugenics (Glenna, Gollnick and Jones, 2007). They noted that the course inclusions were not discretionary decisions by lone faculty members, but approved curriculum by board members.

Additionally, the researchers noted that the land-grant schools disseminated eugenic information to the local community through cooperative extension programmes, one of the eugenic aims promoted by the Eugenics Record Office (ERO) (Glenna, Gollnick and Jones, 2007).

Threat of Black medical professionals

The Progressive Era white supremacists witnessed a rise in emancipated Black people who critically engaged with their existence in the US. Black academics created sociological schools of thought (Morris, 2015), organised political parties and pioneered in the sciences, proving that intellect was bestowed upon all races (Litwack and Meier, 1988). Within 30 years of the end of the Civil War, successful political campaigns for equal rights by Blacks and their white supporters resulted in the ratification of three amendments to the US Constitution, guaranteeing freedom, citizenship and voting rights for the formerly enslaved. Blacks rejoiced at the opportunities to assume civic responsibilities and contribute to the national expansion goals, foremostly, expanding the educational opportunities for their community.

The historical rise of the modern medical professional began during this time. The mid-nineteenth-century medical profession was fraught with 'mutual hostility among practitioners, intense competition, differences in economic interest, and sectarian antagonisms', which resulted in the inability to '[mobilise] its members for collective action or of winning over public opinion' (Starr, 1982: 80). One unresolved issue was the failure of physicians to 'establish clear boundaries marking off members of the profession from untrained and "irregular" practitioners', who, as noted by a European physician who visited the US in 1874, could receive a medical diploma after studying for two weeks (Starr, 1982: 80–81).

The Progressive Era was a time filled with apprehension for all doctors because of the financial insecurity of the profession.

To remain viable, physicians extended their services to veterinary medicine, dentistry, nursing and mortuary sciences (Starr, 1982: 85). To maintain their status and elevate their profession, elites conspired to eliminate those practitioners in the lowest ranks; by strategy, they 'succeeded in shaping the basic organization and financial structure of American medicine' (Starr, 1982: 7–8).

Models of exclusion

Initially buoyant with hope for their future, Black professionals experienced a slow retraction of their dreams for political and social equality. Still reeling from their Civil War defeat and fears of financial destitution, seething Southerners capitalised on several social factors to reassert their authority over Blacks and protect their economic advantages. First, supportive federal government representatives, weary from racial battles and eager to unite the nation, decommissioned the reconstruction bureaus that were created to ease the transition from slavery to freedom for Blacks. Then, the US industrial revolution diverted attention to the creation of national wealth, global status and power.

White supremacists utilised legal and violent means to re-establish the racial hierarchy, including separate-but-equal doctrines, disenfranchisement and domestic terrorism on Black community members. These federal, state and local systems of policies and statutes, eventually labelled Jim Crow laws, served to oppress the meritocratic aspirations of Blacks until the Civil Rights Movement of the 1960s. The American Medical Association (AMA) system of de facto policies extended the oppression to Black medical professionals.

American Medical Association

The AMA is the largest organisation of doctors and medical students in the US. Founded in 1847, the group members established the first national code of medical ethics and have continued to influence medical education, scientific research, and public health policy.

Racist ideology heavily influenced this scientific community. The 1850 AMA third annual conference proceedings presented Dr Samuel G. Morton's research findings that Black people were an inherently different species from whites (AMA, 1850). When some members of the AMA challenged these theories, such as the abolitionist and AMA ethical code committee chair, John Bell, 'sectional discord' was highlighted within the medical field (Baker et al, 2008).

Another source of discord was the exclusion of Black physicians from the AMA. Some white association members believed that scientific qualifications should have been the sole criteria for membership and others 'vehemently opposed associating with Black physicians, either professionally or socially' (Baker et al, 2008: 307). However, the association members were able to bridge their philosophical and sectional differences for the good of the organisational goals, 'teach[ing the divided nation] charity and forgiveness' after the Civil War (Baker et al, 2008: 307).

In the attempt to establish a unified national association, the leaders created an effective policy – the devolution of membership criteria to the local association chapters – to quell heated debate regarding the admittance of Black physicians into the society. With this policy, white supremacist association leaders, particularly but not solely in the southern region of the US, had the political power and professional support to bar Black physicians from membership. 'By the twentieth century, exclusion from these societies often meant professional isolation, erosion of professional skills, and limitations on sources of income' (Baker et a., 2008: 307).

Carnegie Foundation influence

Under the leadership of President Theodore Roosevelt, a Nobel Peace prize recipient who feared white 'race suicide' without eugenic interventions, Congressional representatives symbolically legitimised the Carnegie Foundation for the Advancement of Teaching (CFAT) in 1906 by enacting a charter. The CFAT was just one of the organisations established and funded by the Scottish-born Andrew Carnegie, the well-regarded industrialist and philanthropist. Investigations of the relationship between his wealth accumulation, charitable contributions and social capital revealed that Carnegie had 'few rivals' (Harvey et al, 2011); before his death in 1919, the steel magnate donated an estimated $350 million, or the equivalent in 2019 to £4.2 trillion, to charities (Columbia University Rare Book and Manuscript Library, 2020).

A few key stakeholders in CFAT were white supremacists. Charles Eliot, Harvard University president and American Eugenics board member, reviled the Morrill Acts' purpose of educating poor and Black students as a 'demoralizing use of public money' (Williams, 1991: 67). Woodrow Wilson, Princeton University president and soon-to-be US president, stated 'Negro rule under unscrupulous adventurers (during Reconstruction) had been finally put an end to in the south, and the natural, inevitable ascendency of the whites, the responsible class, established' (Pestritto, 2005: 45), ensuring as president, the racial segregation of federal government offices. Former president of the renamed Case Western University, Charles F. Thwing, fulminated in his book on Australian racial purity that 'the less worthy partner, personal or racial, transmits his character rather than the more worthy one … the dark [skin], rather than the white color persists in offspring … the lower associate pulls down the higher' (Thwing, 1923: 248).

These racially biased, powerful men who represented the upper echelons in the public, private and voluntary sectors of industry garnered material and human resources to fortify the higher education institutions and establish university standards throughout the nation, the academic prestige hierarchy. One of the greatest examples of this influence was the 'Medical education in the United States and Canada: A report to the

Carnegie Foundation for the Advancement of Teaching', also known as the 1910 Flexner Report.

The purpose of the Flexner Report

During the time of incredible national expansion and the emergence of professionalism, the zealousness of the university, professional association, political, philanthropic and religious representatives to develop the best universities in the world was both admirable and fearsome. As intimate partners, they strategically created the modern university system with government and private funds; dictated campus locations; and determined curriculum design. The medical discipline was an area of concern, as it was observed that the university departments desperately needed robust medical school curricula, state-of-the-art medical facilities and technically advanced research laboratories. These elements were considered paramount to the creation of a first-class university system (Flexner, 1910a). Abraham Flexner was commissioned by CFAT in 1908 to appraise the departments of medicine in North America.

The 'failing up' of Abraham Flexner

The AMA conducted its own study of medical schools in 1906. However, to reduce the perception of a biased project, the association recruited Henry S. Pritchett, president of the CFAT, to arrange another study. Because he had 'no expertise' in the medical field, Abraham Flexner was chosen to conduct the evaluation of medical schools. Pritchett somehow believed the lack of knowledge would allow Flexner greater objectivity[3] (Schindler, 2007: 2). Flexner graduated from Johns Hopkins University with a Bachelor of Arts in Classics, which included literature, language, art, philosophy, history based in the North African, Roman, Greek settings. Flexner attended universities in England and Germany, without obtaining an advanced degree (Flexner, 1908; 1930). Throughout the study 'Flexner also enjoyed the promised cooperation of the Council on Medical Education of the AMA, particularly the advice of two of its members, throughout the study' (Wheatley, 1988: 47–49; Schindler, 2007: 2).

Mark D. Hiatt (2000) questioned the methodology used by Flexner in his evaluation of 155 medical schools, particularly the logistics involved in conducting such a mammoth study. In his autobiography, Flexner admitted to possessing a 'sketchy notion' of medical institutions and no foundational knowledge of medicine, yet, only devoted one month to literature review before embarking on the tour across two countries (Flexner, 1960: 5–6; Hiatt, 2000: 1).

Based on calculations of his 1909 field notes, Hiatt concluded that Flexner's schedule across the northern continent via trains, was untenable as only eight months out of 16 allotted for visits were actually utilised. Additionally, the pace claimed by Flexner allowed for just a day or less of evaluation for each medical department, during which he was charged with assessing medical school enrolment; faculty training; endowment size and allocation; laboratory facility and faculty quality levels; as well as, school and hospital relationships (Hiatt, 2000; Siler-Holloman, 2020: 113). Despite the assertion that his findings were high quality, Flexner admitted that he had no standardised data collection method, however, the '"[i]nconsistency never bothered [him]"' (Flexner, 1960: 6–7; Hiatt, 2000: 3). These findings leave doubt as to Flexner's ability to conduct analysis of the medical schools without proper facility data or access to university personnel. Yet, in the introduction of the 1910 report, Prichett assured the reader that the 'accurate and detailed information' in the report had been compared with the data and findings of the American Medical Association and verified by independent observers (Flexner, 1910b: viii).

The CFAT representatives were pleased with the Flexner report. Based on the findings, financial contributions for university medical departments and associated hospitals identified as inadequate either increased substantially or were withdrawn. Using narrative to justify the changes and placate those most affected, Pritchett beseeched the medical school stakeholders and medical professionals to develop educational and professional 'patriotism'; Pritchett explained that the ascription of patriotism required 'loyalty of duty', honesty, 'intelligent sincerity', 'scientific accuracy', 'high ideals' and honour (Flexner, 1910b: xiii).

Impact of Flexner on HBCU medical schools

In the years after the report was published, five Black medical schools 'disappeared', and by 1923 only Howard and Meharry medical schools remained (Duke University Medical Center Library and Archives, n.d.). Flexner graciously advised that the two medical schools were necessary to train Black physicians to work exclusively in the Black community; however, Flexner believed the curriculum should concentrate on public health training rather than surgery (Flexner, 1910c: 180):

> The negro [doctor and nurse] is perhaps more easily 'taken in' than the white; and as his means of extricating himself from a blunder are limited, it is all the more cruel to abuse his ignorance through any sort of pretense. A well-taught negro sanitarian will be immensely useful; an essentially untrained negro wearing an M.D. degree is dangerous. Make-believe in the matter of negro medical schools is therefore intolerable. Even good intention helps but little to change their aspect.

The Flexner Report excluded the effects of classism, sexism and racism in the Progressive Era. However, in his study about the fates of Black medical schools, Earl H. Harley recounted several questionable issues that may have led to the closures. Noting that most HBCUs were managed by white administrators, one institution employed a director with unverified medical qualifications; another suffered from 'lax entrance requirements, lack of academic rigor, poorly qualified faculty and inadequate physical plants' (Harley, 2006). While Harley, and other scholars, realised that the Flexner report did adversely affect the HBCU medical schools, the author believed it was necessary to honestly discuss historical 'failures' within the institutions, learn from them, and apply the lessons to the preservation of the current Black schools (Harley, 2006).

The HBCU medical schools and hospitals provided enriching environments for the development of Black physicians, nurse and other medical professionals. As Black students and physicians were typically excluded from enrolment in white medical schools and from rotations in the white hospitals, they were also excluded from the latest technologies, mentorships and collaborative networks. Marginalisation thwarted their careers. The Flexner Report cemented in place a Black medical education and healthcare delivery system that was separate, unequal, under-resourced, and destined to be insufficient to meet the needs of African Americans nationwide.

Healthcare repercussions of the Flexner Report

Upon the opening of HBCU medical schools, the number of Black physicians rose from 909 in 1890 to 3,495 in 1920 (Savitt, 1987: 10–11). In 2018, Black doctors numbered 45,534 (AAMC, 2021). Though these statistics may seem to show an acceptable growth, when used to calculate the percentage of physicians within the Black population, the results are startling. In 1920, Black doctors represented 3.4 per cent of the total Black community of 10,403,131 persons (Hunt, 1921: 15); by 2018, the percentage dropped to 0.11 per cent of an estimated 42,564,000 Black population (US Census Bureau, 2018). Clearly, the representation of Black physicians has been regressing since the closure of the HBCU medical schools. Even still, the implications of a meagre 4 per cent increase in

Black doctors over 120 years shows that the policies based on the Flexner Report were effective (Ly, 2021).

Despite the doubling of life expectancy of Black people between 1900 and 2010 (Hahn, 2020: 387), Black community members observed macro level medical bias and experienced micro level racial discrimination within the healthcare system (Hamel et al, 2020). Years of mistrust and dismissal may be why less than half of the Black population plan to get the vaccine (Funk and Tyson, 2020). Two doctors revealed many of their colleagues share vaccine hesitancy with their Black patients, contending that their 'white coats do not eradicate our own concerns of mistreatment and disparity' (Okorodudu and Okorodudu, 2021: 229).

After more than a century since the Flexner Report, after a century of technological advances within the elite universities, after the matriculation of the millions of highly intelligent and skilled persons from the highest levels of society, why is the US healthcare system so flawed. Or does the system operate exactly as planned?

Conclusion

The COVID-19 pandemic has served as a litmus test of the US healthcare system. Through the lens of Critical Race Theory, we investigated the vaccine reticence within the Black community, focusing on the historical forces and policies of the Progressive Era. We contended that distrust in the current medical system was attributed to concerted efforts by historical representatives of educational, political, economic and social institutions to preserve their dominant status within the fledgling medical industry. Black inferiority and academic prestige hierarchy narratives served dual purposes to inform, unite and motivate dominant social groups, while deceiving, excluding and inhibiting Black medical education and professionalism. As a counter-narrative, we presented our analysis of the complex relationships between these institutions, myths and the COVID-19 vaccination reticence in the Black community.

Black people in the Progressive Era may have lacked the political, social and economic power to ensure their health and wellbeing. However, today, they have the analytic tools to uncover the racist patterns within the medical industry and use their voices to challenge unproductive and unhealthy narratives. The remaining medical HBCUs, Meharry Medical College and Howard University College of Medicine, have a heavy burden as they continue their mission of educating, increasing Black representation in medicine, and contributing to national policy. As HBCUs have done for over a century, they will take these challenges in their stride, like the noble institutions they have become.

Notes

[1] We are challenging the use of 'minority' when examining phenomenon related to Black and Brown people, as this terminology masks the depth and breadth of related issues.

[2] Within the last year, the topic of Critical Race Theory has garnered strong opposition from far-right politicians and academics.

[3] ' "Failing up" is a contemporary colloquial term that has recently been added to the English Urban Dictionary; to "fail up" means "to derive gain in spite of failure that would usually either preclude said gain or have adverse consequences" ', https://www.urbandictionary.com/define.php?term=failing%20up.

References

AAMC (2021) *Diversity in Medicine: Facts and Figures 2019*, Washington, DC: Association of American Medical Colleges.

Allen, G.E. (1983) 'The misuse of biological hierarchies: the American Eugenics Movement, 1900–1940', *History and Philosophy of the Life Sciences*, 5(2): 105–128.

Allen, G.E. (1986) 'The Eugenics Record Office at Cold Spring Harbor, 1910–1940: an essay in institutional history', *Osiris*, 2: 225–264.

AMA (1850) *The Transactions of the American Medical Association*, Philadelphia, PA: T.K. and P.G. Collins, pp 1–499.

Association of Public and Land-Grant Universities (2019) 'Council of 1890s Institutions, Council of 1890s Institutions', *aplu.org* [online]. Available from: http://www.aplu.org/members/councils/1890-universities/council-of-1890s-institutions.html

Baker, R.B. et al (2008) 'African American physicians and organized medicine, 1846–1968', *Journal of American Medical Association*, 300(3): 306–314. doi: 10.1001/jama.300.3.306

Barth, B. (2010) 'Racism', *European History Online* [online]. Available from: http://ieg-ego.eu/en/threads/europe-and-the-world/racism http://ieg-ego.eu/en/threads/europe-and-the-world/racism

Burk, R.L. (2010) 'Salus erat in sanguine: Limpieza de sangre and other discourses of blood in early modern Spain', *Penn Libraries* [online]. Available from: https://repository.upenn.edu/cgi/viewcontent.cgi?article=1399&context=edissertations

Collins, R. (2019) *The Credential Society*, Chichester, NY: Columbia University Press.

Columbia University Rare Book and Manuscript Library (2020) 'Philanthropy of Andrew Carnegie', Columbia University Rare Book *and* Manuscript Library [online]. Available from: https://library.columbia.edu/libraries/rbml/units/carnegie/andrew.html

Duke University (n.d.) 'LibGuides: Black History Month: a medical perspective: hospitals'. Available from: https://guides.mclibrary.duke.edu/blackhistorymonth/hospitals

Duke University Medical Center Library and Archives (2021) 'Black History Month: a medical perspective: education', Duke University Medical Center Library and Archives [online]. Available from: https://guides.mclibrary.duke.edu/blackhistorymonth/education.

Flexner, A. (1908) *The American College: A Criticism*, New York: The Century Co.

—— (1910a) Introduction by Henry S Pritchett, *Medical Education in the United States and Canada*, New York: Carnegie Foundation for the Advancement of Teaching.

—— (1910b) *Medical Education in the United States and Canada, Bulletin Number Four*, New York: Carnegie Foundation for the Advancement of Teaching.

—— (1910c) *Medical Education in the United States and Canada (The Flexner Report), Carnegie Bulletin*, Boston: D.B. Updike, The Merrymount Press. doi: 10.1001/jama.1943.02840330031008

—— (1930) *Universities: American, English, German*, New York: Oxford University Press.

—— (1960) *Abraham Flexner: An Autobiography*, New York: Simon and Schuster.

Freeman, A.D. (1995) 'Legitimizing racial discrimination through antidiscrimination law: a critical review of Supreme Court doctrine', in K. Crenshaw et al (eds), *Critical Race Theory: The Key Writings That Formed the Movement*, New York: The New Press, pp 29–45.

Funk, C. and Tyson, A. (2020) 'Intent to get a COVID-19 vaccine rises to 60% as confidence in research and development process increases', Pew Research Center [online]. Available from: https://www.pewresearch.org/science/2020/12/03/intent-to-get-a-COVID-19-vaccine-rises-to-60-as-confidence-in-research-and-development-process-increases/

Galton, D.J. (1998) 'Greek theories on eugenics', *Journal of Medical Ethics*, 24: 263–267. doi: 10.1136/jme.24.4.263

Galton, F. (1904) 'Eugenics: its definition, scope, and aims', *American Journal of Sociology*, 10(1): 1–25.

Glenna, L.L., Gollnick, M.A. and Jones, S.S. (2007) 'Eugenic opportunity structures: teaching genetic engineering at US land-grant universities since 1911', *Social Studies of Science*, 37(2): 281–296.

Hahn, R.A. (2020) 'Survival in adversity: trends in Mortality among Blacks in the United States, 1900-2010', *International Journal of Health Services*, 50(4): 387–395. doi: 0.1177/0020731420925289

Hamel, L. et al. (2020) 'Race, health, and COVID-19: the views and experiences of Black Americans. San Francisco, CA' *KFF* [online]. Available from: https://www.kff.org/racial-equity-and-health-policy/report/kff-the-undefeated-survey-on-race-and-health/

Harley, E.H. (2006) 'The forgotten history of defunct Black medical schools in the 19th and 20th centuries and the impact of the Flexner Report', *Journal of the National Medical Association*, 98(9): 1425–1429.

Harris, C.I. (1993) 'Whiteness as property published', *Harvard Law Review*, 106(8): 1707–1791.

Harvey, C. et al (2011) 'Andrew Carnegie and the foundations of contemporary entrepreneurial philanthropy', *Business History*, 53(3): 424–448. doi: 0.1080/00076791.2011.565516

Hiatt, M.D. (2000) 'The amazing logistics of Flexner's fieldwork', *Medical Sentinel*, 5(5): 167–168.

Holloman, T. (2019) *The HBCU Black Woman Professor and the Academic Prestige Hierarchy*, Leeds: University of Leeds. Available from: http://etheses.whiterose.ac.uk/26954/

Hunt, W.C. (1921) *Population, 1920*, Washington, DC: United States Department of Commerce | Bureau of the Census.

Jaynes, G.D. (1986) *Branches Without Roots: Genesis of the Black Working Class in the American South, 1862–1882*, New York: Oxford University Press.

Jordan, W.D. (1968) *White Over Black: American Attitudes Toward the Negro, 1550–1812*, Baltimore, MD: Penguin Books Ltd.

Lee, R. and Ahtone, T. (2020) 'Land-grab universities', *High Country News* [online]. Available from: https://www.hcn.org/issues/52.4/indigenous-affairs-education-land-grab-universities

Leonard, T.C. (2005) 'Eugenics and economics in the Progressive Era', *Journal of Economic Perspectives*, 19(4): 207–224.

Linnaeus, C. (1758) *System Naturae*, London, UK: Forgotton Books.

Litwack, L. and Meier, A. (eds) (1988) *Black Leaders of the Nineteenth Century*, Urbana; Chicago: University of Illinois Press.

Ly, D.P. (2021) 'Historical trends in the representativeness and incomes of Black physicians, 1900–2018', *Journal of General Internal Medicine:* 1–3. doi: 10.1007/S11606-021-06745-1

Morris, A.D. (2015) *The Scholar Denied: W.E.B. Du Bois and the Birth of Modern Sociology*, Oakland, CA: University of California Press.

Norrgard, K. (2008) 'Human testing, the Eugenics Movement, and IRBs', *Nature Education*, 1(1).

Okorodudu, D.O. and Okorodudu, D.E. (2021) 'An issue of trust – vaccinating Black patients against COVID-19', *The Lancet*, 9(3): 228–229. doi: 10.1016/S2213-2600(21)00002-3

Pestritto, R.J. (2005) *Woodrow Wilson and the Roots of Modern Liberalism*, Lanham, MD: Rowman & Littlefield.

Plato (n.d.) *The Republic*, edited by B. Jowett. Adelaide, South Australia: University of Adelaide.

Reilly, P.R. (2015) 'Eugenics and involuntary sterilization: 1907–2015', *Annual Review of Genomics and Human Genetics*, 16: 351–368. doi: 10.1146/annurev-genom-090314-024930.

Reuter, E.B. (1945) 'Racial theory', *American Journal of Sociology*, 50(6): 452–461.

Rollock, N. and Gillborn, D. (2011) *Critical Race Theory*, London: British Educational Research Association.

Savitt, T.L. (1987) 'Entering a white profession: Black physicians in the New South', *Bulletin of the History of Medicine*, 61(4): 507–540. Available from: https://www.jstor.org/stable/44442130?seq=1&cid=pdf-

Schindler, S. (2007) *The Transformation of American Medical Education: The Flexner Report*, Durham, NC: PublicAffairs, pp 1–4.

Seager, H.R. (1913) 'The minimum wage as part of a program for social reform', *Annals of the American Academy of Political and Social Science*, 48: 3–12.

Siler-Holloman, L.A. (2020) *Scholars or Sharecroppers? A Critical Race Historical Exploration of HBCU Black Male Professors*, Leeds: University of Leeds. Available from: http://etheses.whiterose.ac.uk/28671/

Starr, P. (1982) *The Social Transformation of American Medicine*, e-book: Basic Books.

Supreme Court (1927) *Buck vs Bell, Superintendent of State Colony Epileptics and Feeble Minded*, US Supreme Court. Available from: https://www.law.cornell.edu/supremecourt/text/274/200

Tai, D.B.G. et al (2021) 'The disproportionate impact of COVID-19 on racial and ethnic minorities in the United States', *Clinical Infectious Diseases*, 72(4): 703–706. doi: 10.1093/cid/ciaa815

Thwing, C.F. (1923) *Human Australasia*, New York: Macmillan.

US Census Bureau (2018) *The Black Alone Population in the United States: 2018*, Washington, DC: US Census Bureau.

Wheatley, S.C. (1988) *The Politics of Philanthropy: Abraham Flexner and Medical Education*, Madison, WI: University of Wisconsin Press.

Williams, R. L. (1991) *The Origins of Federal Support for Higher Education: George Atherton and the Land-Grant College Movement*, University Park, PA: Pennsylvania State University Press.

FOUR

Pregnancy, pandemic and protest: critical reflections of a Black millennial mother

Sharon Anyiam

This chapter takes an auto-ethnographical approach to understanding the impact of the 2020 COVID-19 pandemic and Black Lives Matter protests on Black millennial resistance. This emerged from my doctoral research into Black millennials and their observations and responses to Black criminalisation and resistance. It will analyse my journal entries, reflecting on my thoughts and feelings towards being a pregnant Black woman during a global pandemic, and the parallel of the international Black Lives Matter protests.

I reflect on my positionality as a researcher and the 'subject' of research. Using two of my journal entries during lockdown, one during pregnancy and the other after childbirth, I will explore how racial justice protests during the pandemic reveal Black millennials willingness to shatter institutional racism. Generating auto-ethnographic research on Black millennial resistance during the pandemic acknowledges and validates

Black millennials' perspectives of resistance. This discussion builds on the scholarly discourse of Black resistance in Britain through the lens of a Black millennial mother.

> Mimi ni a mother. Mimi ni a daughter. Mimi ni a wife. Mimi ni a activist. Mimi a PhD student. Mimi ni a millennial. Mimi a Black woman.

In January 2020, I visited Kenya with the Racial Justice Network to engage with local activists and academics on decolonising education. During one of our workshops, one of the energisers said this phrase 'Mimi ni' which means 'I am' to introduce who we were to the space. The use of this Swahili phrase to declare who we were was a powerful affirmation in the attempt to decolonise our language and the space. Often Black people are othered and criminalised, but in the effort to decolonise the academy and redress epistemic injustices caused by a white supremacist society, the stories and experiential knowledge of Black people must be valued, including their languages. Scholarly work on critical race pedagogy and education has utilised auto-ethnographies to draw attention to epistemic injustices reproduced in educational structures often embedded in white supremacy (Chavez, 2012; Hancock, Allen and Lewis, 2015). Therefore, this chapter is grounded in the critical race methodological practice of amplifying the voices of marginalised groups and acknowledging forms of knowledge not typically valued within academic discourse.

There are no rigid boundaries as to what year(s) of birth individuals had to be born in to be considered a millennial; nevertheless, a majority of researchers mark the beginning of the group in the early 1980s. Brown (2017) marks millennials as the generation born between 1982 and early 2000s, but acknowledges these boundaries are not concrete (Dimock, 2019). Often millennials are misconceived as 'lazy, entitled, selfish and shallow' (Brown, 2017; Stein, 2013). This misconception is extremely dangerous for Black millennials who are more likely to be viewed as deviant than their white counterparts. Williams and Clarke (2018) draw attention to the hypercriminalisation of Black youth through the misuse and over-use of the term 'gang'. As the subject of this chapter, my perspective and experiences of racism in Britain as a Black millennial is vital to understanding the motivations behind Black millennial resistance and mass protests during a global pandemic and lockdown.

Hancock and Allen (2015: 4) note that for auto-ethnographic research it is important to 'name, explain and describe the storied environment' as the context of research frames the narrative. Thus, the contexts that frame my journal entry are the COVID-19 pandemic and BLM international protest, which have yet again brought to the forefront disproportionate health inequalities and police brutality experienced by Black people. Various reports and headlines highlighted that those in the 'BAME/BME' category are most likely to be exposed to the virus and are more likely to die from the virus. This is compounded with the fact that the health status of BAME groups are adverse as they generally have worse health than the overall population (POST, 2007). In a survey of self-reported experience of patients from Black and minoritised groups, Black groups responded less positively to questions about 'access and waiting' or to 'better information and more choice' (DoH, 2009). This conveys a healthcare system that fails to meet the needs of Black people. Furthermore, preceding the murder of George Floyd in the US, police violence and the over-policing of Black communities in Britain has been a current feature (Keith, 1993; Owusu-Bempah, 2017). Scholarly discourse on Black resistance in the UK frequently stresses how institutional racism within policing and the criminal justice system has adversely impacted the relationship between the police force and Black communities, especially Black youths (Elliot-Cooper, 2017; Scott, 2018). This culminated in the widespread protests that occurred in 2011 following the killing of Mark Duggan by the Metropolitan Police.

Furthermore, racism in Britain has also impacted the health status of Black and Brown communities. A report on the youth justice system in England and Wales conducted in 2016 (Taylor, 2016: 2) found over 40 per cent of children from BAME backgrounds, and more than one third, have a diagnosed mental health problem. Additionally, this figure may be higher as it has also been found that individuals from these backgrounds 'are less likely to have mental health problems or learning difficulties identified upon entry to the justice system' (Mental Health foundation, 2019). One of the most startling of these is the mortality rates of Black mothers and infants. This racism that permeates British institutions has been a long-term pandemic affecting the health of Black groups through state-sponsored violence and inadequate health resources and access for BAME groups.

While every generation of Black people living in the UK has experienced racism and criminalisation, the experiences of Black millennials have often been compounded with institutional colour-blind racism. The COVID-19 crisis presents an entirely different component to understanding the racism and criminalisation experienced by Black millennials. The next section will present my reflections of being pregnant and becoming a new mother amid COVID-19 and international BLM protests.

Auto-ethnographic entry

In this section I will present two of my journal entries that explore my reflections in COVID-19 lockdown during and post pregnancy.

During pregnancy

> If someone had told me I'd be experiencing my first pregnancy during a pandemic which would see me restricted to the boundaries of my house in my third

trimester, I would have responded with an equally ridiculous hypothetical situation. But here I am 8 months pregnant and in lockdown! As a Black woman with asthma, COVID-19 already presents a scary thought that I may make up yet another number in the 'BAME' statistics. As a pregnant Black woman with asthma, I'm fearful I may also be yet another number in the statistics of Black mothers who experience inadequate care due to the systemic racism that plagues our healthcare system. When I first found out I was pregnant it felt surreal to envision myself as a mother, but not as surreal as my current reality – one overcome with anxiety about the health of my baby and I. Yesterday I saw headlines about the death of a Black pregnant woman due to contracting COVID-19. She was a nurse at the same hospital my mom works at and was also due to give birth around the same time as me. In her story, I saw elements of my own story. So how can I bring myself to read the story of her death? I cannot even bring myself to vocalise my fears of dying before I get to meet my baby to my family and friends. I do not want to hear that everything will be fine, and I'll be okay, because no one can guarantee me this certainty. No matter how much certainty I seek, what I am about to embark on will be full of uncertainty and I know I must learn to manage my anxieties around these uncertainties. However, doing this whilst being aware of the grim reality that faces Black women during childbirth and the challenges that face Black mothers raising a Black child in a racist world is tiresome.

I don't want to be another story of a Black woman failed by the NHS.

I want to meet my baby.

Post-pregnancy and during protest

As I sit here expressing milk for my today 3-week old baby, it is my brain that is engorged and requires expressing. I'm so thankful my baby made it into the world safely and I got to experience childbirth without complications. Having feared the worst as I approached my due date, I find comfort in the fact my nightmares never became my reality. Yet I have brought my child into a world where the nightmares of Black and Brown people are everyday realities. As my dreams come true and the world greets my child, the world remains in a nightmare state as we mourn the loss of many Black and Brown people to COVID-19 and the loss of George Floyd at the hands of the police. In a time where I feel the happiest I have ever felt, I also feel the immense sadness of witnessing the death of many Black people due to racism. My tears stain my bunched-up top settled across my chest connecting my motherhood to the sorrows of being Black. Finding that tears were rolling from my eyes just as I was about to pump made me even sadder as yet again it was brought to the forefront of my mind that one day I'd have to explain to my child that being Black can be dangerous.

I went to the supermarket alone yesterday for the first time since giving birth. Whilst this may not sound like a big deal for many, it was for me. It felt like a moment of freedom, where I was not worrying if my baby was okay or was not worried I wouldn't be able to cope with normal life things after becoming a mother. This feeling of freedom was short lived as I was followed around the store for 'looking suspicious'. I was the only Black person in the store so it was not a surprise to me that to the white gaze I could look suspicious as I stood in the baby aisle staring at sterilising tablets. When I asked one of the sales assistants if she was following me, I think I shocked her because she mumbled and just disappeared. When the security guard turned up behind me and asked in that familiar Yorkshire tone – 'you alright love?' and I responded, 'am I being followed?'

She told me someone has said I looked suspicious. I did not know how to react. I paused to think of the most appropriate way to respond and all I could muster up was 'that's so ridiculous because I know that someone was your colleague'. I told myself not to make a big deal of the situation as maybe I did look suspicious as I had been standing in one spot for a while and I wanted to go home to my baby without any further delay. As I left the store and the guard looked at me and I was reminded how suspicion has been enough to get Black people killed so I turned to the guard and said something along the lines of, 'with everything going on now you still felt comfortable following the only Black person in the store' and shook my head as I walked away. As I got into my car and drove off it felt like I had just been sprayed by a skunk! The experience left me feeling like I had a bad smell lingering around me. The fact that the security guard chose to follow me rather than watch me over the CCTV was her way of letting me know of her presence and power over me. The aim may have been to deter me from stealing but instead the fact that as the only Black person in the store, standing somewhere for too long made me look suspicious made me feel helpless.

Discussion

The mortality rates of Black women and infants in the UK is reflected in my journal entries as the knowledge of this was a source of my anxiety towards the later stages of pregnancy. A report into maternal deaths in the UK found that there is a 1 in 2,500 chance of death for Black women, which was five times higher than the rate for white women (MBRRACE-UK, 2018). Studies have also shown Black women feel they are not often listened to when they experience pain during labour, which may lead to further complications (*ibid*). My awareness of this systematic racism heavily weighed on my pregnancy during a global pandemic, especially with the high number of deaths amongst BAME groups (Brewis, 2020). The invisibility and silencing of Black pregnant women may potentially be exacerbated by a global pandemic in which prevention measures tend to have been prioritised over the needs of pregnant women. This underlines the importance of giving voice to those who are marginalised, as there are many lessons that should have been learnt from the adverse health status of Black and Brown communities prior to COVID-19 and lockdown. Despite my determination to not make up the statistics of pregnant Black woman who had experienced complications during childbirth, the killing of George Floyd has served as a reminder that the hypervisibility of Blackness in a racist society can be fatal, pregnant or not.

Tate (2016) highlights the struggle to identify racism's invisible touch, which speaks to my experience as a Black millennial. While standing in one place for a long time may appear suspicious, there is no doubt that my visible Blackness was also an unspoken reason why I looked suspicious. It is possible to understand how the widely publicised police and state violence may deter many from speaking up in situations where they feel criminalised. However, the killing of George Floyd and public discourse following his death emboldened me to speak up. Responding to the security guard was an act of resistance, despite risking being portrayed as the 'angry Black woman', the need to give voice to my grievances in a predominantly white space outweighed the risk. Doharty (2020: 548) pinpoints, 'that the stereotypical, racialised controlling images regarding Black women are not exclusive to African-American women and this has led some, in education, to draw on epistemologies such as Critical Race Theory (CRT) because of its usefulness in illuminating patterns of racial discrimination and structural disadvantage'. Thus, in the tradition of CRT, including the narratives of Black millennials furthers our understanding on Black resistance during times of national crisis.

Conclusion

Like a pandemic, racism also kills, and Black millennials have watched digital spaces being infiltrated with violent videos and images of Black and Brown bodies being killed. While social media is full of many Black millennials retelling their stories of racism and criminalisation, there are relatively few accounts of Black millennials speaking of their experiences during the pandemic. The journal entries reflect how the worries and fears of living in a supposed colour-blind racist society were heightened by COVID-19. However, it also highlights the resilience embodied by Black millennials and how their acts of resistance are born from experiencing and witnessing racism and criminalisation before, during and beyond a global pandemic. Moreover, the period of lockdown due to COVID-19 presented a moment of stillness that enabled many to hear and engage with the Black Lives Matter protests. The resistance of Black millennials is the latest narrative of the Black freedom movement that needs to be told. Giving voice to the experiences of Black millennials during the COVID-19 pandemic will enrich our understanding of how the power of individual agency can challenge institutional racism.

References

Brewis, H. (2020) 'COVID-19 cases to be tracked by ethnicity amid disproportionately high number of BAME deaths', *Evening Standard*, 18 April [online]. Available from: https://www.standard.co.uk/news/uk/bame-COVID19-cases-ethnicity-coronavirus-medical-chief-scandal-a4417921

Brown, D. (2017) 'The Gig Economy', SAGE [online]. Available from: https://businessresearcher.sagepub.com/sbr-1863-103233-2807569/20170626/the-gig-economy?download=pdf

Chávez, M.S. (2012) 'Autoethnography, a Chicana's methodological research tool: the role of storytelling for those who have no choice but to do Critical Race Theory', *Equity & Excellence in Education*, 45(2): 334–348.

Department of Health (2009) 'Report on the self-reported experience of patients from black and minority ethnic groups', Gov.uk [online]. Available from: http://www.dh.gov.uk/dr_co nsum_dh/groups/dh_digitalassets/documents/digitalasset/dh_ 100471.pdf

Dimock, M. (2019) 'Defining generations: where Millennials end and Generation Z begins', *Pew Research Center*, 17(1): 1–7.

Doharty, N. (2020) 'The "angry Black woman" as intellectual bondage: being strategically emotional on the academic plantation', *Race Ethnicity and Education*, 23(4): 548–562.

Elliot-Cooper, A. (2017) 'The struggle that cannot be named: violence, space and the re-articulation of anti-racism in post-Duggan Britain', *Ethical and Racial Studies*, 41(14): 2445–2463. doi: 10.1080/01419870.2017.1367020

Hancock, S., Allen, A. and Lewis, C.W. (eds) (2015) *Autoethnography as a Lighthouse: Illuminating Race, Research, and the Politics of Schooling*, Charlotte, NC: IAP.

Keith, M. (1993) *Race, Riots and Policing*, London: UCL Press.

Mental Health Foundation (2019) 'Black, Asian and Minority Ethnic (BAME) communities', *Mental Health Foundation* [online]. Available from: https://www.mentalhealth.org.uk/explore-men tal-health/a-z-topics/black-asian-and-minority-ethnic-bame-communities

MBRRACE-UK (2018) 'Saving lives, improving mothers care', *Oxford Population Health NPEU* [online]. Available from: https://www.npeu.ox.ac.uk/mbrrace-uk/presentations/saving-lives-improving-mothers-care

Owusu-Bempah, A. (2017) 'Race and policing in historical context: dehumanization and the policing of Black people in the 21st century', *Theoretical Criminology*, 21.

Parliamentary Office of Science and Technology (POST) (2007), 'Ethnicity and Health', Parliament.uk [online]. Available from: https://www.parliament.uk/documents/post/postpn 276.pdf

Scott, S. (2018) *The War on Gangs or a Racialised War on Working Class Black Youths*, London: The Monitoring Group.

Stein, J. (2013) 'Millennials: the me me me generation', *Time*: 20: 1–8. Available from: https://time.com/247/millennials-the-me-me-me-generation/

Tate, S.A. (2016) '"I can't quite put my finger on it": Racism's touch', *Ethnicities*, 16(1): 68–85. doi: 10.1177/1468796814564626

Taylor, C. (2016) *Review of the Youth Justice System in England and Wales*, London: Ministry of Justice.

Williams, P. and Clarke, B. (2018) Disrupting the 'single story': collective punishment, myth-making and the criminalisation of racialised communities. In *Racism, Crime and Media*, edited by M. Bhatia, S. Poynting and W. Tufail. Basingstoke: Palgrave.

FIVE

It's alive! The resurrection of race science in the times of a public health crisis

Jon E.C. Tan

Beginnings

The Chinese city of Wuhan, in Hubei province, is 5,474 miles distant from my place of work, Leeds, England. It is the sort of distance that would usually make one feel remote, disconnected and removed from the lives of the 11 million inhabitants in this far-off city. That is probably how many felt in the UK, and other parts of Europe and the West, when news of a new strain of coronavirus (denoted as COVID-19 or SARS-Cov-2) was reported in Wuhan in December 2019. Distant, remote, isolated – words that often make up our language of defence, separation and irrelevance. We use these words as protection against those things that we feel may put us in some sort of jeopardy. How many times do we hear the phrases, 'I'd keep your distance', or 'it's an isolated incident', or even 'It's not something remotely relevant?' They are words that both describe distance and *create* distance.

With a name like 'Tan', you may have already guessed that I have a Chinese heritage. In fact, I can trace my cultural connections through English towns, Welsh valleys, and Chinese shorelines. I am British-born, yet I stand at the confluence of these three cultures. So, when COVID-19 appeared in Wuhan, although physical distance remained, in other, cultural ways, I felt more closely involved (perhaps perilously so). You see Wuhan is only 700 miles from my Chinese, ancestral beginnings in Guangdong province, roughly 100 miles less than the journey between John O'Groats and Land's End in the UK. Passing through the province of Hunan, the fast train from Wuhan to Guangzhou makes a breathtaking journey of only four hours.

Early coverage of the situation in Wuhan by Western media also prompted a cultural resonance within me. There seemed a lot of images of the food markets of the region – busy, bustling places. Without listening to the words of such reports, the images brought back childhood memories of visits to various places where my family then resided, mainly in Malaysia, Singapore and Hong Kong. In Sabah, I remembered the markets down by the shoreline, where the day's catch would be brought directly from a myriad of small, colourful fishing boats to the market stall (that is, if you had not chosen 'your' fish as it lay in the boat). In the heat of the day, stall-keepers would draw down an awning and sleep in its protective embrace. By night, the markets would become places to eat. Night restaurants where the rich colours were a vast array of produce I saw during the day, were transformed into a barrage of sensory experiences. In Hong Kong too, the street restaurants that opened in the evening were places where a rich cultural tapestry was painted, where 'Westerners' mingled with China and the East with a great familiarity born from hundreds of years of association. East meets West. In Tsim Sha Tsui, Mong Kok, Sha Tin, Sham Shui Po, and from Kowloon Tong to the floating restaurants of Aberdeen harbour, it was real, your senses told you so. Through sight, sound, taste, smell, these were ways through which our human experiences became enriched. Absorbing these spaces, this was my ethnography, long before I knew the meaning of the word.

Looking back, these places were ones of fusion, of meeting, of sharing. They existed as such in my experiences in so many different ways. Most of them had a colonial past and, at some point in their history, could be prefixed as one of those British Territories Overseas – a strange phrase that suggests places, people, communities, nations and land can be possessions and property; that one nation, so far distant, can have dominion over another. It was still British Hong Kong when I was a child, and on the way there I still flew into British Royal Air Force stations in Cyprus and the Maldives. The reach and legacy of Empire. On visits back to family in Malaysia, my father reminisced about his own upbringing; we played football in the grounds of his English Catholic school and talked of the English Tea House in the hills above the town. At other times we swam in the sparkling, clear waters off the island of Berhala, where, during the Second World War, another imperial power, Japan, had established a prisoners of war camp for captured Allied servicemen, mainly British and Australians. East meets West.

I tell you all this to let you in, so that perhaps we can be a little closer as I tell the story of a global pandemic taking hold, and my growing anxieties about how communities and cultures were portrayed, how racism and the long reach of race science fuelled discourses of difference, distance and distrust. It is a story of power, the exercise of it, the fear of losing it, the way it manifests in different forms. Perhaps, most importantly, it is one of long-standing racism focused on Chinese-Asian communities, amplified in times of crisis, of which the global COVID-19 pandemic is one in a long line of examples.

The pandemic (and racism) take hold

11 March 2021: I write something brief in my work diary, for today marks the first anniversary of the World Health

Organization's (WHO) declaration of the COVID-19 crisis as a global pandemic. In their Situation Report 51, they then documented, globally, 118,319 confirmed cases of the virus and 4292 deaths (WHO, 2020). I take a moment to reflect, glancing outside from the home-based 'office' that has been my fixed abode for the last 12 months. Through my window to the outside world, I spot my neighbour putting his refuse bin out. I wave and he waves back in acknowledgement. Here in the UK, we are still in 'lockdown' in our government's attempts to combat infection. This is the third such period where all but essential services have been closed. While there is a glimmer of hope with immunisation getting underway, taking stock of where the world is now is by no means heartening. In the week that most children in England began returning to classrooms, the weekly briefing from WHO (2021) recorded more than 116 million cases and over 2.5 million deaths worldwide, with the most persistent increases being recorded in Europe and the Americas.

With my family spread wide across the globe, I naturally scan WHO (2021) updates for the individual countries in which they reside. Let me get this straight: I am not one for the assemblage of neoliberal league tables and I did not approach my comparison of countries in this way. Instead, I felt compelled to thinking about risk and the relative safety of my relatives. I have Chinese cousins in Malaysia, Australia and North America, as well as in China, so I scroll through the official data tables to these places. I am struck by the disparities. It is with some relief that I see that in Malaysia there has been just over 963 cases and 3.6 deaths per 100,000 people. In China too, the figures show even smaller numbers of cumulative cases and deaths per 100,000 (6.9 and 0.3 respectively). I call one of my cousins in Melbourne and, although now out of many of their restrictions on movement, I sense that lockdown has also been challenging. Humour has always been our ways of coping with tough times and, in between the laughter, we both catch a glimpse of the realities, the loneliness, the repetitive soullessness of each day, the juggling of keeping a job, keeping a home, keeping the home schooling going. I return to the WHO (2021) report, finding some comfort to know that Australia has similar cumulative statistical returns as Malaysia. Concern for relatives elsewhere is not alleviated by the figures and I feel sick to my stomach as I read and reread the numbers for North America and for the UK. Why is it so much worse here? As I write, the US has recorded over 28.6 million cumulative cases. That is over 8,641 cases per 100,000 people. There have been more than 519,000 deaths (156.8 deaths per 100,000). I hope my family in San Francisco and friends in New York and Rochester are safe. The Americas as a whole, make up 48 per cent of the total of recorded COVID-19 deaths, with Europe contributing a further 34 per cent. In the UK, over 4.2 million cases and almost 125,000 mortalities to date are documented by WHO (2021). Looking back, by these indicators the situation in China is hugely overshadowed by the UK's 6,206 cases and 183.3 deaths per 100,000 of the population.

If there was any relief gained from my consultation of these global comparisons, it is short-lived. The figures make for sobering reading. Behind every statistic, a story of suffering. For many, an agonising, suffocating death. I have seen close loved ones, specifically my English grandmother and Welsh grandfather, lose battles with respiratory conditions. Certainly, the vulnerabilities of age and underlying health conditions have become familiar, dominant concerns since the beginning of the pandemic. Yet, my anxieties are not confined to such parameters. Although science and policy strategy has continued to express its main concerns with its focus firmly fixed on them, I have greater ones about race and health inequalities and of the surge in racism directed against Chinese and Asian communities.

The first reported cases of COVID-19 in the UK were recorded at the end of January 2020 (Weaver, 2021). The case involved a Chinese family that had travelled from Hubei province in support of their son, a student starting a new term at the University of York. They stayed in a hotel and did a little sightseeing. It is amazing what hindsight affords us, but we have to be careful not to judge any individual actions too quickly. At this point, when the family travelled, China had recorded only one death related to COVID-19. Wuhan and Hubei province were yet to be locked down. There seemed little indication as to the virulence of this strain of coronavirus. Here in the UK, the Prime Minister, Boris Johnson, delegated the chairing of the first emergency meeting (COBRA) to his Health Secretary, Matt Hancock. Throughout most of January 2020, the risk level in the UK was considered low, with Public Health England (PHE) and the Department for Health (DfH) moving the official classification from 'very low' to 'low' on 22 January 2020. Thinking back to the ways in which the UK government (and its advisory group, SAGE) talked about the developing situation, I am amazed at how relaxed it all feels. It is dismissive, a language of remoteness, of distance. The image of one of those 'Keep Calm and Carry On' posters from wartime Great Britain flashes into my head! Such a thought is not as random as one might think: Prime Minister Johnson is a biographer of Winston Churchill and wartime rhetoric seems to be his 'go to' stock of phrases and sentiment. It is as if he is rallying the troops; perhaps the podium outside 10 Downing Street should be replaced by a Willys jeep, so that he can engage in his oratory, standing on its bonnet! Yet, perhaps Boris is less Churchill and more Shakespeare's Richard II, missing the warning in John O'Gaunt's words. No more:

> this scepter'd isle,
> This earth of majesty, this seat of Mars,
> This other Eden, demi-paradise,
> This fortress built by Nature for herself
> Against infection and the hand of war
>
> (Shakespeare, 1988: 388)

Indeed, a sleepy England chose to tread slowly in its response to the unfolding crisis. While it chose a language that suggested its fortress defences against infection were prepared, incidents of anti-Chinese, anti-Asian racism were spreading rapidly like a brushfire. As early as February 2020, the British mainstream press was reporting significant increases in acts of violence, abuse and hatred against Chinese communities (Campbell, 2020). By May, police data showed incidents of anti-Chinese/Asian racism in the first two months of the year to have outstripped figures for the whole of 2019 and 2018. A pandemic of a different kind was awakening.

Anti-Asian racism: the resurgence of an old problem

So far, it had been a glorious day. The sun had shone all the way up to London, as we attempted to calm our excitement about being out of class for our school History and Science trip – our destinations being the British Natural History and Science museums on Gloucester Road, South Kensington. The best part of the morning had been spent in among the bones of dinosaurs, of huge whales and other mammals, then to the smallest of skeletons of birds, bats and marsupials. Walking the corridors of that awe-inspiring architectural wonder that is the British Natural History Museum, we encountered vast collections of taxidermy, of creatures great and small, even some extinct. As a child still of school age, this array of 'things', of 'stuff' was overwhelming. London was not unfamiliar to me, as my father had friends here that we visited – people that he had been friends with as a member of the Chinese student community. During these family excursions, I had seen other collections of 'stuff': The British Museum, on Russell Square; The Victoria & Albert Museum. It was now lunchtime and our teachers called us together to sit in groups, in the gardens. I reached into my rucksack for the food my mother had packed for me. There was a packet of crisps and, oh, a small chocolate biscuit. Fabulous! Better still she had avoided making those cheese and tomato sandwiches that, on a previous school trip, had become all soggy, as the tomato juice bled into the bread.

Instead, my parents had baked some small parcels of pastry, filled with a Malaysian-type curry. They were gorgeous and I broke one in half to start eating. 'Errr, what's that?', came a voice. 'Curry', I said, 'D'ya want one?' 'That's disgusting, err, I'm gonna vomit', came another voice. 'Is it cat or dog?', questioned another. Others joined in; others stood by. Teachers just seemed preoccupied with getting us to the next part of the visit. For me it was not the first, nor last, time that I felt racism.

Anti-Chinese and anti-Asian racism are nothing new. From full-blown anti-Chinese riots in American and British cities in the late 1800 and early 1900s, through discriminatory legislation in the US, to acts of violence, verbal abuse, property-damage and killings, racism towards the Chinese community in the 'West' has been commonplace. Yet, it has been poorly documented and reported, largely due to the community being silent and more likely to deal with such hostility internally. That suggests some level of mistrust within the community that crimes against them will be properly investigated by those in authority (Adamson et al, 2009). The work by Sue Adamson et al (2009) is one of very few pieces of published research that has attempted to shed light on the incidence of anti-Chinese/Asian racism in the UK. Even in what we might now call a pre-COVID-19 world, the report makes for worrying reading, suggesting that the Chinese communities in the UK are one of those most likely to experience racially motivated abuse and to be victims of similarly motivated hate crimes. As they summarise:

> [T]he report reveals that the Chinese community suffers from levels of racism that are not only unacceptable but also, given the prevalence of under-reporting within the Chinese community, that there are perhaps even higher levels of racial violence or harassment than those experienced by any other minority group. This view is contrary to the established myth of the Chinese being a satisfied community that is immune from

racism. Additionally, the lack of adequate reporting in the gathering of official statistics, possibly itself driven by stereotyping, means that the real picture remains unacknowledged. Even when Chinese victims persist in reporting race crimes, including serious offences, they frequently face a response that is shaped by institutional racism – a state of inaction and denial.

(Adamson et al, 2009: 10)

I read through the summaries of the types of victimisation, from the ever-present verbal abuse to the physical attacks. Then the loss of livelihoods through businesses targeted by arsonists, to the loss of life, following a beating from a gang. Sadly, there is nothing surprising in what I read; plenty of it a lived experience. A feeling of disembodiment comes over me as I cast my academic analytical eye over my past experiences. Conversations that I would overhear in my school: 'Did ya hear about X? He went up to the Chinky [Chinese takeaway] again and keeps asking them for Alsatian and chips.' There was always laughter surrounding these moments, even when it was someone reporting on how their local Chinese takeaway or restaurant had, once again, had its windows smashed. It was not my laughter, but sometimes it included my British friends – remember I was not British to them, at least not in the same way. 'Fucking hate them smelly, Chinkies, me', I would hear, followed by one of my more clued-up friends quizzically stating, 'hold on, Jon's Chinese'. The response from the perpetrator of the racial slur, at least in this supposed 'safe space' for me, was always, 'yeah but Jon's different, he's alright'. I learned to avoid violence. I learned of safe places and no-go areas. I learned routes home. I learned what to protect my family from. In school, I learned that mediocrity in class performance did not attract attention. I learned silence.

Almost 40 years have passed since those personal experiences. There have been incidents that have punctuated my adult life too. Time, as distance, is perhaps some insulation from them, but it is a fragile protection. Now, as I read and listen to daily updates on the COVID-19 crisis, it is apparent that the pandemic has given rise to an unhealthy environment in which anti-Chinese and anti-Asian racism has flourished. In Europe, the phenomenal increases in such racism have been well documented by researchers such as Wang et al (2020). At the same time, these studies have clearly shown how circumstances brought about by the pandemic have highlighted long-standing injustices perpetrated against these Asian communities. As Wang et al (2020: 17) writes:

> During the COVID-19 pandemic, people of Chinese origin in France from different backgrounds – especially in terms of age and migratory status –, are raising their voices against racism. While for recent young immigrants racism can be perceived as a new topic, for other Chinese descendants and earlier immigrants it is more deep-rooted. Thus, activists of Chinese origin may conceptualize their struggle as anti-racism, as a movement for agency in society which is sometimes combined with the anti-racist struggles of other Asian-perceived people and other people of colour, as well as struggles for other issues related to gender, sexual identity, etc.

In the UK, where incidents of anti-Chinese/anti-Asian racism have increased three-fold in a matter of months (Campbell, 2020), writers such as Matt Detzler are keen to point out that the pandemic has seen the mobilisation of the Right in attempts to normalise anti-Chinese/anti-Asian racism into the mainstream. As he documents, such racism is seen in the spread of conspiracy theories, linking COVID-19 to the actions of China as a state (Detzler, 2020) and in the assignations by even some mainstream media that COVID-19 was manufactured in a state-funded laboratory. I sense a mistrust of China in the majority of 'Western' reports about COVID-19 specifically, and China more generally. Sudworth's report for the BBC in June 2020 (Sudworth, 2020) is a good example of how all activities by China surrounding the virus and its investigation are presented as suspicious and questionable. Moreover, its conclusions, that transmission from animals to humans were more likely a 'natural spillover event', are presented in ways that suggest this is a peculiarly Chinese, cultural problem. Later reporting on the outcomes of the WHO inspections in Wuhan similarly seek to cast doubt upon the independence of the WHO inspectors' findings and suggest the official pressure from Chinese authorities have resulted in a conveniently favourable outcome for China (BBC, 2021b). Even in the reporting of a WHO inspector's defence of the report, Chinese cooperation and the integrity of the research, mainstream media can be seen re-enforcing the position that China should remain under suspicion (BBC, 2021a).

Examining this rhetoric of suspicion, one has to engage with the significant anti-Chinese position adopted further west in the US (Dhanani and Berkeley, 2020). The historical and institutionalised racism against Chinese communities in the US is well known. What is interesting is the parallels we can draw between historical events such as the fears and prejudices that resulted in the acts of violence against the Chinese community in San Francisco in the July 1877 riots and subsequent anti-Asian immigration laws and controls. As argued by Risse (2012), the anti-Chinese/Asian position adopted by the US in pre-1904 America marks the intersection of racism, historical intergenerational fears of mass infections, and the economically-driven and politically-motivated othering of Chinese/Asian communities. Certainly, as Risse (2012) documents, these positions follow familiar patterns, for example the portrayal of these communities as immigrants; threatening the employment of white workers; of communities growing out of control; as being sources and spreaders of disease; and being morally dubious. From my 2021 standpoint, I note a similar coincidence of racism, economics and negative portrayals of Chinese culture in the speeches of the US President, Donald Trump, at the time of the COVID-19 outbreak. Coupled with his general isolationist, anti-immigration stance, and his use of the word 'plague' to describe COVID-19 (there was a bubonic plague outbreak in San Francisco in 1877), I cannot help feel the weight of these racialised, historical continuities.

Zoonotics, virological origins and the science of blame

31 March 2021: I switch on the television as I eat my lunch. Today, the Minneapolis policeman, Derek Chauvin, is in court for the first day of witness testimony, in which he stands accused of the murder or manslaughter of George Floyd. He denies all charges. The words of the witnesses and the video footage of Floyd's life ebbing away, as Chauvin knelt on his neck, are powerful and traumatic. The public killing of this African American man in May 2020 gave rise to a global outcry and demonstrations, turning a spotlight on institutional and structural racism. It was a moment when people of colour, including Chinese communities, felt solidarity in their shared lived experiences (Anand and Hsu, 2020; Wang et al, 2020).

In other news today, I note the publication of the UK government's inquiry into 'race and ethnic disparities' (CRED, 2021) – a governmental commission, set up in the wake of the Black Lives Matters demonstrations in the UK, following the events in Minneapolis, Minnesota. I cannot help feel a sense of contradiction, denial and a recasting of responsibility in this document. The report seems to suggest claims of institutionalised racism can be explained away by other more credible data (for example, social class; income; family culture). There is then a huge number of recommendations that suggest things at institutional levels need to change. How can a country and its institutions 'be regarded as a model for other white-majority countries' (CRED, 2021: 10) when so much needs to be done to tackle inequalities that exist, at the very least, on intersectional lines that include race as a factor?

The language of the report emphasises what the evidence shows, separating it from what might be perceived and felt. It is a very classical position in the establishment of knowledge, but the careful words of Ryan (2006) resonate within me as I read the Commission's evidential claims: 'Critics of positivist epistemologies have insisted that divisions between objectivity and subjectivity, or public and private knowledge, or scientific and emotional knowledge, are socially constructed. Just as important, these artificial divisions, or dualistic ways of viewing the world, are used to control ideas about what knowledge is legitimate' (Ryan, 2006: 16). Conversations about research span many years of my professional life, and one in particular comes to mind: that for raw data to become evidence it needs the application of a process of interpretation. In the construction of 'what this means' and in the resultant effect of such an interpretation on an audience's understanding, this is where the science gives legitimacy to ideological beliefs, hidden or otherwise. As argued by Saini (2019) and Evans (2019) the legitimisation of race as a concept, race as an explanation of difference and as a justification for different treatment, exploitation and oppression has been greatly served by science and its institutions.

A similar reliance on the scientific community to present the world with seemingly objective, dispassionate, apolitical knowledge has been very evident throughout the COVID-19 pandemic. Scientists have shared official podiums with government; they have been at the heart of decision-making. We have gotten to know the names of epidemiologists, virologists and public health advisers on a countrywide and worldwide scale. Their role in tracking the daily progress of the virus and the response of science in the development and implementation of vaccines has been indisputably important. However, perhaps in other ways, science and the emphases placed on the origins of the coronavirus outbreak have fuelled anti-Chinese, anti-Asian racism. At the centre of this is the way in which the scientific narrative has been constructed; the dominant way in which we are persuaded to make sense of the pandemic almost exclusively through an epidemiological lens.

As Klingberg (2020) argues, a virus alone does not make for a pandemic. In understanding how quite common localised outbreaks of a virus become a more serious global crisis, epidemiology alone provides a very limited explanation. Instead, one has to consider the wider 'existing social, ecological, and political relationships ... [in the] the transformation of a local disease outbreak into a pandemic' (Klingberg, 2020: 367). By this, Klingberg (2020) and other researchers have emphasised that these conditions are not exclusive to China, but are a product of globalised economics, urbanisation and the march of global capitalism. Such warnings are not new. We find such concerns, for example, in Smith et al's (2007) discussions of global disease and in Aguirre's (2017) consideration of biodiversity loss and the heightened risks of zoonotic transmission, whether we consider outbreaks of Ebola in Africa or H1N1 in Central America. In this sense, there is a global responsibility for the COVID-19, SARS-Cov-2 pandemic in ecological, economic and behavioural terms. Furthermore, part of a virus becoming a pandemic must lie with the capacity of a global community and individual nation states to respond accordingly. Looking back to the WHO (2020: 1) update, I spot their concerns of 'alarming levels of inaction' and as I think over the data returns that show disproportionate infection and death rates among people of colour and those living in impoverished, crowded conditions. I hang my head. As Phan and Wood (2020) document, a significant part of this public health and economic catastrophe has been ill-preparation and prioritisation in public services for a known risk.

Instead, the use of science has focused on the origins of the zoonotic event that has served political purpose to suggest the singularity of source and conditions, culturally specific to China. As politicians, Western media and the institutional apparatus for knowledge production have taken this up. The resurgence and reinvigoration of anti-Chinese, anti-Asian racism has become an inevitability. As Klingberg (2020: 367) summarised:

> The weaponized idea of a 'Chinese virus' requires the illusion of a single origin point as well as the illusion of isolated local responsibility. The Huanan Market in Wuhan offered international news reports the setting for an imagined zoonotic event, where a bat virus latent in a 'wild' animal jumped to humans because of the racist notion that (all) Chinese eat such things (see Pan 2020). There are certainly some in China who do eat exotic animals, but this is neither a cultural characteristic nor commonplace.

Conclusion: recolonialism, power and fear under the cover of a global catastrophe

Throughout the world and across the centuries, colonial expansion, its holding power and its justification of privilege, has been well served by the social and scientific construction of race (Saini, 2019). In particular, the activities of 'Western' science enabled a discourse of superiority to become established as a powerful 'truth'. This 'truth' told us that particular groups of people were morally and intellectually inferior; that their customs, beliefs and social practices were strange and uncivilised; and that it was, therefore, a right (God-given in most cases) and act of humanity for those deemed superior to hold dominion over them. Places, people, communities, nations, and land could legitimately become property, possessions, subject to a higher power. Most importantly, the discourse enabled cultural riches and economic wealth to be carried away, perhaps in ways so guilt-free that great cities and their architecture could be built, almost in celebration of such piracy. Statues to those most successful in these endeavours could be erected and collections of things could be 'preserved' in national museums. Race science facilitated the expansion of an economic and cultural agenda. Such colonialism was not the sole preserve of the 'West', but it set in motion a global competition that required difference, not common humanity, to be emphasised.

As I look back at the last 12 months and the rise of anti-Chinese, anti-Asian racism, I cannot help but wonder whether such phenomena are not simply a product of the COVID-19 pandemic. A more general rise in racism and isolationist, nationalistic sentiment has followed the global economic crisis of the second decade of the twenty-first century (Elias et al, 2021). Certainly, the pandemic has amplified such positions. Perhaps, then, as some Western nations become nervous of their global economic position and seek to make themselves 'great again', and to 'build back better', the resurrection of science, utilised racially in gaining a perceived advantage, is unsurprising. Thus, while current cases of animal-to-human transmissions in 2020–2021 are seen as the result of a kind of cultural barbarity that is the sole preserve of China, its people and government, other such incidents of zoonosis and the activities of governments in playing them down are conveniently forgotten. As Best (2001) reminds us, Western governments and, particularly those of the UK and US, acted to misinform, deny and distract when Bovine Spongiform Encephalopathy (BSE) first appeared in British cattle in 1986. It was ten years before the then British Secretary of State for Health, Stephen Dorrell, reluctantly announced that the source of the human variant of the disease (Creutzfeldt-Jakob Disease, nvCJD) was linked to BSE, and had entered the food chain through encouraged industrial practices and relaxed governmental policies and actions.

In such moments, perhaps the greatest fear is of losing power, influence and economic advantage on the international stage. As globalised economies seek to recover and jostle for more favourable positions, the continued ambivalence in relations between Western and Eastern players, once again, comes into sharp relief. If responsibility for the outbreak and development of SARS-Cov-2 into a worldwide pandemic is sought, then it is a collective one, with those great exponents of marauding global capitalism taking the spotlight. A dominant discourse that emphasises China's part over and above that of this, more global, responsibility, may then tell us more of the ideological processes through which the recolonialisation of economic spaces as virtual territories becomes justified. What is clear is that racism at all levels is, once again, a purposeful, persistent and characteristic centrepiece in this political and economic opportunism.

References

Adamson, C.B., Craig, G., Hussain, B., Smith, L., Law, I., Lau, C., Chan, C.K. and Cheung, T. (2009) *Hidden from Public View? Racism Against the UK's Chinese Population*, London: Monitoring Group London Civil Rights & Arts Centre.

Aguirre, A. (2017) 'Changing patterns of emerging zoonotic diseases in wildlife, domestic animals, and humans linked to biodiversity loss and globalization', *ILAR Journal*, 58(3): 315–318.

Anand, D. and Hsu, L.M. (2020) 'COVID-19 and Black Lives Matter: examining anti-Asian Racism and anti-Blackness in US education', *International Journal of Multidisciplinary Perspectives in Higher Education*, 5(1): 190–199.

BBC (2021a) 'COVID: UK scientist defends WHO fact-finding mission to Wuhan. COVID: UK scientist defends WHO fact-finding mission to Wuhan', *BBC News*, 14 February [online]. Available from: https://www.bbc.co.uk/news/world-asia-china-56061879

—— (2021b) 'Coronavirus: more work needed to rule out China lab leak theory says WHO', *BBC News*, 31 March [online]. Available from: https://www.bbc.co.uk/news/world-asia-china-56581246

Best, S. (2001) 'Cows, capitalism, and cover-ups: the politics and economics of mad cow disease', *Tamara: Journal of Critical Postmodern Organization Science*, 1(1): 31.

Campbell, L. (2020) 'Chinese in UK report "shocking" levels of racism after coronavirus outbreak', *The Guardian*, 9 February [online]. Available from: https://www.theguardian.com/uk-news/2020/feb/09/chinese-in-uk-report-shocking-levels-of-racism-after-coronavirus-outbreak

Commission on Race and Ethnic Disparities (CRED) (2021) 'The Report', Gov.uk [online]. Available from: https://www.gov.uk/government/publications/the-report-of-the-commission-on-race-and-ethnic-disparities

Dhanani, L.Y. and Franz, B. (2020) 'Unexpected public health consequences of the COVID-19 pandemic: a national survey examining anti-Asian attitudes in the USA', *International Journal of Public Health*, 65: 747–754.

Detzler, M. (2020) 'I am not a virus – anti-Chinese racism and coronavirus', *Wales TUC Cymru*, 1 September [online]. Available from: https://www.tuc.org.uk/blogs/i-am-not-virus-anti-chinese-racism-and-coronavirus

Elias, A., Ben, J., Mansouri, F. and Paradies, Y. (2021) 'Racism and nationalism during and beyond the COVID-19 pandemic', *Ethnic and Racial Studies*, 44(5): 783–793. doi: 10.1080/01419870.2020.1851382

Evans, G. (2019) *Skin Deep: Journeys into the Divisive Science of Race*, London: Oneworld Publications.

Klingberg, T. (2020) 'More than viral: outsiders, others, and the illusions of COVID-19', *Eurasian Geography and Economics*, 61(4–5): 362–373. doi: 10.1080/15387216.2020.1799833

Phan, P.H. and Wood, G. (2020) From the editors: doomsday scenarios (or the black swan excuse for unpreparedness), *Academy of Management Perspectives*, 34(4): 425–433.

Risse, G.B. (2012). *Plague, Fear, and Politics in San Francisco Chinatown*, Baltimore: Johns Hopkins University Press.

Ryan, A. (2006) Post-Positivist approaches to research. In *Researching and Writing Your Thesis: A Guide for Postgraduate Students*, Maynooth: MACE.

Saini, A. (2019) *Superior: The Return of Race Science*, London: 4th Estate.

Shakespeare, W. (1988) 'The tragedy of Richard the Second', in W. Shakespeare, *The Complete Works*, Oxford: Oxford University Press. Speech by John O'Gaunt, quoted at p 388.

Smith, K.F., Sax, D.F, Gaines, S.D, Guernier, V. and Guégan, J-F. (2007) Globalization of human infectious disease, *Ecology*, 88(8): 1903–1910.

Sudworth, J. (2020) 'Wuhan: city of silence: looking for answers in the place where coronavirus started', *BBC News* [online]. Available from: https://www.bbc.co.uk/news/extra/ewsu2giezk/city-of-silence-china-wuhan

Wang, S., Chen, X., Li, Y., Luu, C., Yan, R. and Madrisotti, F. (2021) '"I'm more afraid of racism than of the virus!": racism awareness and resistance among Chinese migrants and their descendants in France during the COVID-19 pandemic', *European Societies*, 23(1): S721–S742. doi: 10.1080/14616696.2020.1836384

Weaver, M. (2021) 'Timeline of the UK's first recorded COVID cases last year', *The Guardian*, 26 January [online]. Available from: https://www.theguardian.com/world/2021/jan/26/timeline-of-the-uks-first-recorded-COVID-cases-last-year

World Health Organization (WHO) (2020) 'Coronavirus disease 2019 (COVID-19) Situation Report – 51', *World Health Organization*, 11 March [online]. Available from: https://www.who.int/docs/default-source/coronaviruse/situation-reports/20200311-sitrep-51-covid-19.pdf

—— (2021) 'Weekly epidemiological update', World Health Organization, 9 March [online]. Available from: https://www.who.int/publications/m/item/weekly-epidemiological-update---10-march-2021

SIX

It's just not cricket: (green) parks and recreation in COVID times

Kavyta Kay

One, among many, areas of inequality on which COVID-19 has placed a spotlight is access to green spaces. That the nation's local parks and green spaces have been a lifeline during the pandemic is a widely agreed-upon sentiment; yet while these have been invaluable, the Green Space Index released in 2020 revealed that 2.7 million people in Great Britain do not have access to such a space. Additionally, a survey by Friends of the Earth (2020) found that 42 per cent of people of Black, Asian and Minority Ethnic backgrounds live in England's most green space-deprived neighbourhoods.

If green spaces enable wellbeing practices such as walking, exercising and playing in the park, then the question of who gets to inhabit these spaces invariably arises. Over the course of the pandemic, recreational cricket, a sport widely played by South Asian communities nationwide in these green spaces, was confronted with this question of access. The issue further took on an intersectional dimension as we saw notions of privilege, race and identity collide in particular ways, which is explored in this chapter.

The green space gap

In the digital age of information overload that we are living in, a cursory Google search brings up a plethora of articles on all manner of gaps and inequalities globally – for example the gender pay gap, the racial gaps in educational attainment, labour legislation, health inequalities and so on; all starkly highlighted during the pandemic and set to exacerbate once we eventually navigate a post-pandemic world (International Monetary Fund, 2020). One social cleavage that came under scrutiny in the COVID-19 era was the green space gap, which identifies a correlation between green space deprivation, income and race (Friends of The Earth, 2020). Worldwide lockdowns showed us the extent to which green spaces are invaluable for our wellbeing, both mental and physical, and while this has been an unexpected upside, the disproportionality for those who can access green natural environments and those who cannot became apparent. In recent years, a raft of research has shown that greenness rewards us with positive health outcomes and concepts such as forest bathing, a Japanese form of ecotherapy translated from *shinrin-yoku* (Li, 2018), and green prescriptions (Jorgensen and Robinson, 2020) have become mainstreamed. Yet green spaces arguably are not mainstreamed as one in five people struggle to access them. Recent studies revealed that the global majority live in the most green-space deprived neighbourhoods and are some of the most affected by this shortage (Collier, 2020; Public Health England, 2020) and race becomes a key vector in this disparity. A survey commissioned by the Ramblers (2020), Britain's leading walking charity, revealed that in addition to race, household income was also a significant factor. Only 57 per cent of adults questioned said that they lived within five-minutes' walk of a green space, be it a local park, nearby field or canal path. That figure fell to just 39 per cent for people from a Black, Asian or minority ethnic (BAME) background and 46 per cent for those with a household income of under £15,000 (compared to 63 per cent of those with a household income over £35,000 and 70 per cent with a household income over £70,000). At a juncture when clear connections have been established between structural racism and the impact of COVID-19 on people of colour across the country, the wider-ranging benefits that would come from closing the green space gap would inevitably yield positive outcomes, yet a closer examination of the differential levels of engagement and enablement with green spaces paints a complex, albeit messy, picture. This messy engagement takes on another dimension in the interactions of British Asians,[1] the intricacies of their relationship with green spaces and how this, alongside park cricket as a performance of Brown bodies in these spaces, is closely tied to historical legacies of racism and colonialism.

Unequal by design

Natural England, the British Government's advisory body for the natural environment in England, published the Access to Natural Greenspace Standards, which state, 'local authorities should consider the provision of natural areas as part of a balanced policy to ensure that local communities have access to an appropriate mix of greenspaces providing for a range of recreational need' (2020: 2). What emerges are the questions of how far are these spaces from the residents' homes and how many local authorities implement the standard? Given that local authorities face a different set of pressures to consent to housing developments, the consequence is a pushback on the existing green spaces, with the resident communities trying to defend the few that do exist. The encroachment of developments on green spaces is an issue also felt by recreational cricket.

According to the GMB Union, more than 200 school fields are being sold off across England to build 'affordable' housing (TES, 2019) and the loss of fields and cricket pitches will impact children and young people in damaging ways.

All these statistics illustrate how dimensions of race, class and gender, which will be explored further below, intersect to create social, material and symbolic boundaries in green spaces. Fields in Trust, an independent charity protecting parks and green spaces, state that 'in a difficult economic climate, the provision of parks and green spaces should be prioritised in areas with lower socioeconomic groups and a higher representation of BAME communities given the disproportionately high level of benefits that these groups derive from parks and green spaces' (2018: 8) They go on to state that 'in terms of motivations, BAME groups appear to use their parks and green spaces more socially than those from white ethnic background and that a significantly higher proportion of BAME groups also report using parks and green spaces for team sports (11%) compared to white groups (5%)' (2018: 34). In a COVID-19 climate, certain communities, who are already priced out of mainstream cricket, faced further limitations in terms of access and training facilities during lockdown restrictions. Leisure under lockdown altered socialities across the board, and in the era of social distancing, this emerged as a politicised and racialised issue as different demographics were affected differentially. For example, in July 2020, the reimposition of tier 4 restrictions hours before Eid, particularly in areas of high Muslim populations across northern England, was met with criticism among the British Muslim community, and was largely received as a biased decision metered out to a community that has been continually othered. Additionally, a disproportionate number of fines were handed to Asian and Black communities for breaking lockdown rules (Gidda and Busby, 2020), echoing Nirmal Puwar's (2004: 145) argument that 'marked bodies are under super-surveillance' in that they are treated suspiciously within particular spaces. These are just a few of many obvious examples of systemic racism leading to a broader question of whether the issues faced by the Black and South Asian communities in the 1970s and 1980s, only one generation old, have completely disappeared. Or have they taken on a new form, through microaggressions and invalidations? Or both?

Puwar's ideas can be further understood through an examination of park cricket, which takes place mainly in public green spaces. While formal club cricket laid dormant for most of 2020 and cricket balls declared by the British Prime Minister Boris Johnson a 'natural vector of disease', recreational/park cricket, widely and fervently played by South Asians nationwide, was not only impacted by the pandemic in particular ways but also revealed long-standing sentiments reflective of the legacy of the British Empire.

Until you see yourself represented, you're always going to feel rejected

Sathnam Sanghera wrote:

> From the nineteenth century, the game became innate to empire, the Imperial Cricket Conference's efforts to standardize the rules of the game helping to bring the many disparate parts of empire together, while the values of fair play, courage and resilience, nurtured on the games fields of public schools were seen as key to developing the imperial ruling race.
>
> (Sanghera, 2021: 5–6)

Historian Prashant Kidambi (2019: 1) points out in his opening line on the evolution of cricket during the British Raj, 'If the origins of cricket were decidedly rural, the beginnings of Indian cricket were indubitably urban.' To an extent, many decades later, we see that play out in Britain, with amateur players using up whatever space available to them in built-up urban environments, for example public parks, empty beer gardens, vacant car parks, back alleys, housing rooftops alongside parks and fields.

Green becomes remade into cultural sites for building community identity. 'By a curious historical twist, a sport that defined the identity of the former colonizers is now the ruling passion of the country that they conquered' (Kidambi, 2019: vii). For the first generation of South Asians to settle in Britain arriving as servants, as *ayahs* (nannies), as sailors, as soldiers, as workers, as artistes, as refugees, as visitors, as students, as traders, as carers, identity politics as linked to sport became about 'how South Asianness is nurtured and celebrated through cricket, rather than being a "condition"' (Raman, 2017). For many South Asians, cricket has become a repository for emotional attachments to 'home', through migrant narratives of vindication and empowerment, which are simultaneously a critique of a British polity, which, they feel, continues to racialise and exclude its migrant 'others' (Raman, 2017: 76). Cricket is closely linked to the historical legacies of colonialism, and racism sits at the core of a disjuncture between contemporary British Asian players and mainstream cricket. At a league level, the processes of exclusion of British Asians have been long documented and were thrown into the spotlight during Azeem Rafiq's testimony at a Parliamentary select committee in 2021, of institutional racism he faced at Yorkshire County Cricket Club:

> Whilst cricket has helped ethnic communities to create important social networks at the same times as inspiring diasporic connectivity, this has also served to entrench two types of cricket across the United Kingdom. The first is white, traditional and mainstream, while the second is Asian or Black and very much urban based and deprived of good quality facilities and finance to develop sustainable club structures.
>
> (Holden, 2020)

There is mass Asian participation in cricket on a variety of different levels. From playing the games in their thousands to travelling around the country supporting their 'home' teams, many play for fun, and few become professional players.

In a conversation with Harjot Sidhu, content creator of *London Writing Guy*, a sports blog dedicated to British Asians in cricket, he addresses this:

> those [recreational cricket] were set up as a resistance mechanism to, in a sense to traditional English cricket and this idea of Englishness. Maybe the flouting was a continuation of that, the sense of you can't tell me what to do. The Asian community was victimised right from the off. The 50s, 60s and 70s from having come over here. The National Front stuff and what they had to endure, from colonialism and potentially having their rights stripped of them in that manner, finally having got rid of that in terms of gaining independence and having been invited to the UK, and finally thinking they have an element of acceptance in and realising we still haven't been accepted. There is this element of we've never been accepted, so why should we listen to what the government tells us. We weren't accepted in India or Pakistan or wherever, we came over here and we still weren't accepted. They don't actually care about us so why should we care about them? As Aarti Ratna (2013) echoes, "being 'in' a sporting space is not the same as being 'of' that space.

The racialised emotions that are engendered from othering and exclusion are ones that have long marked British Asian communities and are persistently theorised through a problematic culture-clash framework that connotes homogeneity and a condition of being static (Kay, 2021). Otherness becomes about occupying liminal spaces outside the centre of power, marked by whiteness and embodied by the presiding institutions, and this manifests in the racial performativity within green spaces and sporting spaces, in this case park cricket. This finds resonance with Thomas Fletcher's (2015: 1) statement that 'to this day cricket operates strict symbolic boundaries; defining those who do, and equally, do not belong'. This reinforces the ideological underpinning that certain bodies are entitled to a space and others are not, what Puwar (2004) terms 'space invaders'. British Asians' racialised emotions of rejection are triggered from perceptions as being culturally distinct from the white British norm (Kundnani, 2012), particularly along religious and ethnic lines. These emotions found an outlet in the widespread disagreements around the deployment of the label BAME in early 2020, which had gained significantly more traction in the British media over the course of the pandemic, to discuss the disproportionate impact of the virus on the global majority. It also became a generalising acronym metered out to groups who do not fit the normative white standard, and against the backdrop of protests and a pandemic the frequent utterance of BAME as a referential point, which othered ethnic groups in conversations on equality, diversity and inclusion in its reductive classification, was largely condemned. Othering became further reinforced through hegemonic and homogenising discourses on national identity and exclusionary imaginations of various ethno-religious groups that entered the mainstream during the referendum and Brexit and still continue to date.

The processes of exclusion are not a new revelation. Carrington and Macdonald's (2001:49) study stated that 'racism is both deeply rooted and pervasive in recreational cricket in England'. This racial genealogy of cricket, to a large extent, continues the emotions of acceptance and rejection in which racialised notions of Englishness are deployed to exclude participation of Black and Asian players from the official leagues, and for ethnic minority women who are marginalised on both gender and racial lines, this becomes a more entrenched issue, particularly as they are continually theorised through a 'culture clash' model. The latter, which was mentioned earlier, needs to be updated, as it fails to wholly speak to the multifaceted subjectivities of millennial British Asians. The absence of research on women's experiences in cricket in general already is revelatory in terms of the masculinisation of this sector, and the absence of research on minority women is even more pervasive. The Active People Survey showed that South Asian participation in sport (particularly among Pakistani and Bangladeshi women), falls consistently below other social groups (Hylton et al, 2015: 6)

It is evident that there is a need to examine the dynamics that, over a sustained period of time, have led to Asian women not playing cricket, which Sidhu further relates to the COVID-19 context:

> There will be setbacks everywhere. Where Asian female representation was lagging anyway, it will be setback even further. It comes to ECB potentially investing more in it and capitalising on Asian female role models like Naomi Dattani, the likes of which can have a say in the community. Where women struggle to play or find acceptance in the first place and not being able to potentially train, they might just have simply given up and thought 'may as well get a job'. Where they might have preserved before and where issues of gender inequalities, acceptance and rejection, that year of lockdown may have compounded all of that.

In addition to these, safety emerges as a pressing issue, which Sidhu provides another insight into:

> So if you got 11 or 22 guys and there's a full-on cricket match going on and a woman wants to get involved, I do feel it would be a difficult thing. I can't talk from a female perspective, but I remember speaking to a journalist, Annie Chave. Considering she's a white woman in Somerset, when she was a kid she had to pretend she

was a boy to play cricket. Now if a white woman in a cricket loving area has to do that, it becomes difficult to imagine what an Asian woman going into a park, where there's potentially boisterous guys, how she's going to feel. I think they would be put off and I do think it's a difficult thing for them.

The gendered consequences are being challenged though game drivers such as Shivanie Patel, who started a cricket club to inspire girls and young women in Bradford, and Mina Zahoo, who runs Bolly Cric-Hit, a combination of Bhangra and fitness, combined with softball cricket: "Cricket, especially in the South Asian community, has traditionally not been a game for women and girls but Bolly Cric-Hit has helped change this and given females of the household the chance to participate and enjoy themselves' (ECB, 2020). There is also some movement in the participation of South Asian women in cricket, for example with the 2021 Dream Big Desi Women campaign. While a positive initiative, it is worth considering the gendering of time and labour. For instance, as a consequence of the pandemic, home schooling largely fell on women's shoulders and, consequently, became extra labour mainly borne by women. Therefore, the capacity and time to engage in sport, even at a recreational level, became an unfortunate trade-off. As we continue to live with COVID-19, at the time of writing the take up of cricket for South Asian women remains minimal but, in an increasingly evolving cultural climate, it is hoped that Asian women's participation in this sport will be encouraged and enabled at all levels.

Mighty oaks from little acorns grow

The old English proverb 'mighty oaks from little acorns grow', loosely interpreted as great things can come from small beginnings over time, is a personal favourite, deployed in response to detractors who negate efforts to combat racial and social injustice, be it through social protest, digital activism, or small acts of resistance. Let us relate this to South Asian players. Through informal conversations with South Asian students and those working within the community, a pattern emerged of a public perception of recreational cricket as anti-social, particularly as it is mainly constituted by Black and Asian players. As seen earlier, the questions of where these communities play and what spaces they are 'allowed' to inhabit have continually been contested. A consensus also emerged that most British Asians are priced out of mainstream league cricket due to the heavy cost of training and equipment, as well as cultural barriers to participation. There is great passion and significant involvement at an informal level and recreational cricket could be conceived of as a space of resistance. Off-grid cricket, lying outside of the ECB purview, which takes place in car parks, council-owned pitches and streets are unregulated, is thriving, and we saw that over lockdown, regulations were flouted in the pursuit of the game. On deeper reflection, one could make the claim that the unofficial cataloguing of these games would point to the power that British Asian recreational players have in the future of the game, which could be interpreted as institutional rejection, an arena in which the mechanisms of exclusion, such as casual racism and/or microaggressions and othering, are the norm. Recreational cricket then becomes an alternative and rich space of untapped talent. If one interprets decolonising as an attempt to reverse the legacy of inequality and racism left by colonialism, then perhaps a case could be made that recreational cricket is a decolonial tool. As a student recounted on a Master's course I lead on decolonial thought, race and education:

> Just look at the role of the umpire – their regulations processes and how it excludes people of colour. When you take it to the streets, then you get the full control of it. It doesn't just become then the site of resistance, but it also becomes the site of activism where people literally

take to the streets. Geographically speaking, so much action actually happens there. Because once you're in a building, you're instantly institutionalised. Outside of the institutions, there's something freeing about it.

When one contemplates the variety of cricketing traditions and what underpins these, it is clear it isn't just about cricket.

What do they know of cricket that only cricket know?

This passionate and probing question by eminent Trinidadian writer C.L.R. James taken from his groundbreaking *Beyond A Boundary* (1963), asks of this not just as a sport, but as culture. In this part autobiographical memoir, part appraisal of West Indian cricket, part indictment of colonialism, he calls attention to the embodiment of values and ideas stratified by race and class in the praxis of daily life through cricket. This chapter has illuminated some of the cultural dimensions of cricket through a British Asian lens, and offers a proposition that we are perhaps seeing decoloniality in action through recreational cricket, in which a residual colonial practice is altered to a subversive anti-colonial one.

As it currently stands, the use of recreational cricket as a method of resistance to hegemonic structures is likely to have taken a hit because of the cleavages created through COVID-19 and losing 18 months of practice; opportunities for trials may have taken a backseat due to the economic impacts of the pandemic. Despite the global challenges, recreational park cricket will remain a lifeline for South Asian communities. It continues to be more of a draw than club cricket because of the cultural barriers to participation, as this chapter has explored, and its role in cultivating community spirit is not to be underestimated. The London Cricket Trust, a charity that aims to put cricket back into London's parks through free-to-use cricket nets is a wonderful initiative to increase participation in overcoming the long-standing barriers of associated costs and accessibility. Arguably, though, for these to work optimally, parks and green spaces should be available but, as we saw earlier, deeper infrastructural problems will potentially impact the green spaces. Alongside this, we are also seeing changing attitudes from British Asian communities to the relationship with natural environments in general.

Nature for all?

The surge in popularity of green spaces over lockdown was not only an important moment in recognising the value to our health and wellbeing, and our oneness with the earth, but also challenged dominant modes of thinking, particularly for first-generation Asian migrants to this country, in which progress and modernity was aligned to material urbanism (Collier, 2020) and nature was arbitrary (with the exception of the odd day out, as hilariously depicted in Gurinder Chadha's (1993) comedy *Bhaji on the Beach*). The poet Benjamin Zephaniah posits: 'First and second generation immigrants to Britain experienced racism and for them it was about survival and not going back to rural poverty. Now they want their kids, the third generation, to be much better qualified than the average white guy' (Hoare, 2016).

A study by Natural England found that in 2017, 25.7 per cent of Asian people visited the natural environment and spent time in the countryside compared to their white peers, who came in at 44.2 per cent (Gov.UK, 2017). Another report from the Campaign to Protect Rural England (CPRE) painted a similar picture in its estimation that people from Black, Asian and minority ethnic backgrounds account for about 1 per cent of visitors to national parks. There are manifold reasons as to why this is the case, and research by Sport England (2015) posited six barriers: language, awareness, safety, culture, confidence and perception of middle-class stigma. All of these are highly inflected by race. The Asian community in Britain is not a monolith and, while many of the barriers faced by people from these communities are intersectional, for example socioeconomic status, location, access, gendered spaces where the double yoke of sexism and racism plays out, the natural environment remains widely regarded as a white domain where the threat of hostility and biases looms large, a dynamic that was brilliantly observed by Anita Sethi in *I Belong Here* (2021).

The Glover Report (2019) added: 'We are all paying for national landscapes through our taxes, and yet sometimes on our visits it has felt as if National Parks are an exclusive, mainly white, mainly middle-class club, with rules only members understand and much too little done to encourage first time visitors' (Glover, 2019: 15). One of the earlier academic studies was Chakraborti and Garland's *Rural Racism* (2004), which contextualises issues of racist victimisation in the rural arena, and which could be currently characterised as microaggressions. More recently, Corinne Fowler (2020) offered a creative response in her deconstruction of rural England as a 'white space', and how ethnic minorities are deeply intertwined with the British countryside, traced back from the days of Empire; for example, many of the country houses, woodlands and moorlands were financed either by the slave trade or fortunes made in India through the East India Company. Exclusionary concepts of Englishness are rendered redundant, yet still persist, and any interrogation of this is met with attack. This, in my view, is a mischaracterisation and, if anything, wider inclusion of global majority people in supporting local and national green spaces through a greater understanding of Empire's relationship to the latter, as well as improving our relationship with these environments, will serve everybody for the better in its critical pedagogy. As COVID-19 has highlighted, the importance of higher levels of social responsibility, and a considered application of this care, opens up a new set of possibilities in negating the sentiments of cultural rejection with a less neoliberal capitalist take and a more community-centred approach.

Defending the lungs of our cities has to be a part of every citizen's survival mechanism because we depend on our green spaces, and turning the discussions of access, inclusion and infrastructure into politicised attacks will not have any long-term benefits whatsoever to all sides. By 2050, an estimated 29.7 per cent of our population will be from the global majority. In the words of the Glover (2019) report: 'Our countryside will end up being irrelevant to the country that actually exists.' It is hoped that the new shifts in attitude post-pandemic will yield a more positive approach to the green space gap, as I end with well-known scholar and environmental activist Vandana Shiva's (Atmos, 2020) reflection:

> A relationship with nature is not a relationship of privilege. The revolution of our times – for young people, for old people, for Indigenous people, for everyone – is to take care of the Earth. Find a way, find your little piece of Earth to take care of. And together we can. And together we must.

A personal pandemic postscript

Nature and sport are considered microcosms of society and the public conversations within and across these arenas are indeed a critical reflection of race relations in modern-day Britain. We have seen anti-racism take centre stage in the wake of Black Lives Matter 2020 and End the Virus of Racism[2] 2021. Racial justice initiatives have been deployed across a range of settings, but there is still work to be done, and a long way to go. As we are about to navigate a post-pandemic world, there are some propositions that I would call for:

- That Asian communities in Britain feel excluded and othered at varying levels has been the central premise of this chapter. Sustained engagement with these communities, some of whom may not want to be engaged with, needs

to be initiated in diffuse ways, for example partnering with Asian outlets, promoting cricket trials and community countryside trips/walks to raise awareness.
- Having been forced to examine my own feelings towards the natural environment in the past two years (as someone who had formerly had no interest in it) was a personal and illuminating journey, which led me to consider if I were made aware of conservation career options, my career trajectory might have been different. Community champions and role models in cricket and conservation and sustainability need to be promoted to encourage more participation in these spaces at all levels and to demonstrate these as viable career options, especially for Asian young women across the land.
- Education: In line with the principles of the decolonising curriculum movement, a meaningful teaching unit on the relationship between colonialism and British culture (in the areas of cricket and the countryside, to give just two examples) would certainly go a long way in increasing and improving the current conversations on race in twenty-first-century Britain.
- Access to green spaces for the purposes of recreational and informal cricket has laid bare yet another barrier to British Asian mainstream representation in the sport. As such, intersectional and critical studies to explore the nuances of these relationalities between institutions, communities and landscapes would yield fascinating insights that would be a useful starting point.
- In addition to representation, there needs to be cultural and organisational change at all levels through, for example involving communities of colour in decision-making, demonstrating real engagement and less box-ticking – all with the end goal of making communities feel welcome in these spaces, which currently run counter to what we are seeing in league cricket, in spite of efforts from the ECB with the formation of the South Asian Action Plan in 2018.

- The imbalances in parks and green space participation need to be addressed. Whether to practise a game, to recruit players, to socialise, to meditate, to hike, to heal, to hang out: 'We all need access to nature and open green space as an antidote to the everyday stressors of city living, and not least the anxiety-inducing impact of this COVID-19 crisis' (Collier, 2020). One way of overcoming barriers is to set up groups where people of colour feel safe and comfortable and where cultural provisions can be planned and, in this manner, Asian communities can experience and learn about the great outdoors and the natural environment more widely.

Representation matters. It is very important to have people visible in these spheres who look like you, which then makes activities in the sporting and outdoor worlds not only aspirational, but attainable. This needs to be embedded across all elements of cricket and the outdoors, for example outdoor adventure, sports and walking magazines, and on television, for example on programmes like *Countryfile*. At a development level, representation matters too; for example, fully training South Asian people as community champions, group leaders, or outward-bound instructors is just as important as having access to people who are not from the usual backgrounds. Create opportunities and different avenues for people to reconnect with cricket and the outdoors, which will at the very least encourage South Asians, and the global majority, to participate inclusively.

Notes

[1] This term is employed here for working purposes only, while acknowledging that as an identity category in Britain, it collapses particular class, ethnic and religious identities even if not all British Asians identify as such. While British Asian may be seen as too broad in its encompassing of the diverse cultures emanating from South Asia and erasing difference, and also too narrow in its limited and stereotypical understandings of notions of heritage, tradition and culture, it is a term that has continuing currency in Britain.

[2] Launched following a spike in hate crimes against people of East and South-East Asian descent in the UK since the start of the COVID-19 pandemic.

References

Carrington, B. and Mcdonald, I (2001) *'Race', Sport and British Society*, New York: Routledge.

Chakraborti, N. and Garland, J. (2004) *Rural Racism*, New York: Routledge.

Collier, B. (2020) 'The race factor in access to green space', Runnymede Trust [online]. Available from: https://www.runnymedetrust.org/blog/the-race-factor-in-access-to-green-space.

ECB (2020) 'Women's big cricket month | Your stories', ECB [online]. Available from: https://www.ecb.co.uk/england/women/news/1840617/womens-big-cricket-month-stories

Fields In Trust (2018) 'Revaluing parks and green spaces. measuring their economic and wellbeing value to individuals', *Fields In Trust* [online]. Available from: http://www.fieldsintrust.org/Upload/file/research/Revaluing-Parks-and-Green-Spaces-Report.pdf

Fletcher, T. (2015) 'Cricket, migration and diasporic communities identities', *Global Studies in Culture and Power*, 22: 141–153.

Fowler, C. (2020) *Green Unpleasant Land: Creative Responses to Rural England's Colonial Connections*, Leeds: Peepal Tree Press.

Friends of the Earth (2020) 'England's green space gap' [online]. Available from: https://policy.friendsoftheearth.uk/print/pdf/node/190

Gidda, M. and Busby, M. (2020) 'BAME people disproportionately targeted by Coronavirus fines', Liberty Investigates [online]. Available from: https://libertyinvestigates.org.uk/articles/bame-people-disproportionately-targeted-by-coronavirus-fines/

Glover, J. (2019) 'Landscapes Report', Gov.uk [online]. Available from: https://assets.publishing.service.gov.uk/government/uploads/system/uploads/attachment_data/file/833726/landscapes-review-final-report.pdf

Gov.UK (2017) 'Visits to the natural environment', Gov.uk [online]. Available from: https://www.ethnicity-facts-figures.service.gov.uk/culture-and-community/culture-and-heritage/visits-to-the-natural-environment/latest#by-ethnicity-last-7-days

Hoare, B. (2016) 'Diverse nature: does nature conservation represent society?', Discover Wildlife [online]. Available from: https://www.discoverwildlife.com/people/diverse-nature/

Holden, R. (2020) 'The globalisation of sport and its impact on national identity in England and Wales', in J. O'Brian, R. Holden and X. Ginesta (eds), *Sport, Globalisation and Identity: New Perspectives on Regions and Nations*, Routledge: New York.

Hylton, K., Long, J., Fletcher, T. and Ormerod, N. (2015) *South Asian Communities and Cricket*, Leeds: Yorkshire Cricket Board.

International Monetary Fund (2020) 'Life post-Covid-19' *Finance and Development* [online]. Available from: https://www.imf.org/en/Publications/fandd/issues/2020/06/how-will-the-world-be-different-after-COVID-19

James, C.L.R (1963) *Beyond a Boundary*, London: Yellow Jersey Press.

Jorgensen, A. and Robinson, J.M. (2020) 'Green prescriptions: should your doctor send you for a walk in the park?', The Conversation, 24 July [online]. Available from: https://theconversation.com/green-prescriptions-should-your-doctor-send-you-for-a-walk-in-the-park-143231

Kay, K. (2021) 'Staff and student racial microaggressions in Brown Britain', Revista da APBN [online]. Available from: https://abpnrevista.org.br/index.php/site/article/view/1268/1183

Kidambi, P. (2019) *Cricket Country: An Indian Odyssey in the Age of Empire*, Oxford: Oxford University Press.

Kundnani, A. (2012) 'Multiculturalism and its discontents: left, right and liberal', *European Journal of Cultural Studies*, 15(2): 155–166.

Li, Q. (2018) *Shinrin-Yoku The Art and Science of Forest-Bathing*, London: Penguin.

Natural England (2020) 'Providing accessible natural greenspace in towns and cities' *English Nature* [online]. Available from https://www.google.com/url?sa=i&rct=j&q=&esrc=s&source=web&cd=&cad=rja&uact=8&ved=0CAQQw7AJahcKEwjgor6pqoX8AhUAAAAAHQAAAAAQAw&url=http%3A%2F%2Fpublications.naturalengland.org.uk%2Ffile%2F78003&psig=AOvVaw24ASCwYIEDYMx2Ifn3VH-P&ust=1671527242433732

Patel, K.J. and Shiva, V. (2020) 'A wave of change', Atmos [online]. Available from: https://atmos.earth/kevin-patel-vandana-shiva-climate-interview/

Public Health England (2020) 'Improving access to greenspace. A new review for 2020', Gov.uk [online]. Available from: https://assets.publishing.service.gov.uk/government/uploads/system/uploads/attachment_data/file/904439/Improving_access_to_greenspace_2020_review.pdf

Puwar, N. (2004) *Space Invaders: Race, Gender and Bodies and Out of Place*, Oxford: Berg.

Raman, P. (2017) 'It's because we're Indian, innit? Cricket and the South Asian diaspora in post-war Britain', in T. Fletcher (ed.), *Cricket, Migration and Diasporic Communities*, Oxford: Routledge.

Ramblers (2020) 'The grass isn't greener for everyone: why access to green space matters', *Ramblers* [online]. Available from: https://www.ramblers.org.uk/news/latest-news/2020/september/the-grass-isnt-greener-for-everyone.aspx

Ratna, A. (2013) 'Intersectional plays of identity: the experiences of British Asian footballers', Sociological Research Online [online]. Available from: https://journals.sagepub.com/doi/10.5153/sro.2824

Sanghera, S. (2021) *Empireland: How Imperialism Has Shaped Modern Britain*, London: Penguin.

Sport England (2015) 'Getting active outdoors: a study of demography, motivation, participation and provision in outdoor sport and recreation in England' [online]. Available from: https://sportengland-production-files.s3.eu-west-2.amazonaws.com/s3fs-public/outdoors-participation-report-v2-lr.pdf?_2SJK6Ube9RCSPcrYJD5vxFnGzBSiO5M

TES Reporter (2019) 'School playing fields sell-off criticised', TES [online]. Available from: https://www.tes.com/news/school-playing-fields-sell-criticised

SEVEN

Muslim funerals during the pandemic: socially distanced death, burial and bereavement experienced by British-Bangladeshis in London and Edinburgh

Farjana Islam

Introduction

Since the pandemic surged in the UK, funerals across all religions and secular sectors, for both COVID-19 and non-COVID-related deaths, took on a new character, due to the adherence of necessary social distancing rules. This created added demands and stresses for both funeral service providers and mourners, as funeral directories were struggling to manage an excessive number of funerals, as well as ensuring necessary precautions for the safety of funeral staff. The Muslim religion constitutes the second largest religion after Christianity in the UK; the majority of followers have South-Asian ancestry (Office for National Statistics [ONS], 2011). Funeral rites play a significant role for Muslims, both theologically and socially

(Jahangir and Hamid, 2020); therefore, some families were saddened by the socially distanced funerals and the omission of some rituals that they expected for their beloved ones (Parveen, 2020).

In the UK, 92 per cent of Bangladeshis are Muslim, who in turn constitute the second largest Muslim community in the UK (ONS, 2011). 15 per cent of Muslims in England and Wales are of Bangladeshi descent, which has been one of the worst affected ethnic minority communities during the coronavirus pandemic (PHE, 2020a). Public Health England's (PHE) analysis associated with COVID-19 transmission, morbidity and mortality suggested that British-Bangladeshis had around twice the risk of death when compared to white British people during March to May 2020 (PHE, 2020b: 4). The high death rate of Bangladeshi-heritage people created unprecedented challenges to the funeral and bereavement structures in the UK. These challenges merit special attention considering the impact of COVID-19 on British-Bangladeshi people and their life-transitional services (see Hunter, 2016; Maddrell, 2016; Stevenson, Kenten and Maddrell, 2016).

The disproportionate impact of COVID-19 on the Bangladeshi communities has energised the ongoing discourse on sociostructural inequalities in the UK (Islam and Netto, 2020). The PHE's analysis also concurred that the pandemic exacerbated long-standing inequalities associated with housing challenges and poorer socioeconomic circumstances, which made the Bangladeshi people more vulnerable to COVID-19 infection. The majority of British-Bangladeshis are Commonwealth immigrants who are concentrated in post-industrial conurbations, with about half of them living in London (ONS, 2011). In terms of socioeconomic class, the Bangladeshis are broadly characterised as a post-industrial working class (Watt, 2008), who are undertaking many low-pay, manual, or key frontline[1] jobs, such as transport and delivery, healthcare assistants, and supermarket workers. These types of frontline jobs disproportionately exposed many British-Bangladeshis to virus infection. Moreover, the European immigrants with Bangladeshi ancestry (that is, Bangladeshis who have a dual citizenship with Italy, France, Germany, and so on) might also have been infected disproportionately as they are significantly employed as taxi drivers and chauffeurs, sales and retail assistants and other lower skilled jobs[2] in direct contact with the public (Islam, 2019).

This chapter aims to explore the challenges faced by British-Bangladeshi Muslims in relation to performing funeral and mourning rituals at community level while adhering to social distancing rules. After a brief discussion of Islamic funeral rites and the methodology of this study, the chapter will shed light on some distresses and challenges perceived by Bangladeshi mourners in terms of staging the funerals and bereavement of six men of Bangladeshi heritage who died during the pandemic. The chapter also discusses recommendations based on four informants' reflections to address similar funeral challenges in the future, with a view to providing the appropriate tribute to the Muslim deceased on their passage to their final destination.

British-Muslims' funeral needs: an overview of Islamic rites, rituals and custom

Since the 1980s, Muslim councillors and community leaders have worked with local councils to facilitate Islamic funeral rites in the UK. Therefore, Muslim sections were gradually opened in some public graveyards, specifically in the Greater London area (Maddrell et al, 2018; Afiouni, 2019). Nowadays, public cemeteries in major UK cities have reserved plots for Muslims. Also, there are some Muslim-only private cemeteries across the UK (for example, the Garden of Peace and the Eternal Garden in London). From the beginning of the twenty-first century, repatriations of the deceased person to countries of origin, which was previously idealised for Commonwealth immigrants, underpinned by the notion of the 'myth of return',[3] have significantly decreased (Gardner, 1998).

The creation of multitude burial places in Greater London and other major cities has contributed to setting the trend of Muslim burials in Britain, and thereby the funeral rituals of the British-Bangladeshi community have been increasingly moving from Bangladesh to Britain (Gardner, 1998; Afiouni, 2019).

Muslims believe death is the passage from this world to the afterlife, where the departed soul will continue to live eternally (Cheraghi, Payne and Salsali, 2005). The Prophet of Islam instilled the value of honouring the deceased through a set of funeral rites, which play a significant role for Muslims both theologically and socially (Jahangir and Hamid, 2020). The pertinent funeral rituals include a quick burial, washing the body (*ghusl*), shrouding the body in white clothes, and the funeral prayer for the deceased (*Janazah*) (Jahangir and Hamid, 2020; Maravia, 2020). Although ritual practices are unequivocal in Islam, different groups and nationalities have subtly modified the customs to fit the local culture, social environments and geographical circumstances (Jahangir and Hamid, 2020). Therefore, the expression of grief and mourning varies among different ethnic groups and nationalities in the UK due to blended religious and cultural connotations in their country of origin as well as customs in the UK (for example, burial with a coffin in the UK). The bereavement and mourning practices in Bangladesh are structured on Islamic beliefs, which are also idealised among the British-Bangladeshi communities across the UK. After burial, people visit the bereaved to offer condolences, and neighbours or friends provide food for the bereaved family for at least a three-day mourning period (Yarrington, 2010). The Prophet recommended this practice as an act of virtue and kindness that brings friends and neighbours closer to each other (Reza, 2020).[4]

During the COVID-19 outbreak, the fulfilment of these important Islamic funeral rites was challenging. Some Muslim funeral directories lifted the requirement of washing and shrouding for COVID-19-related/suspected or confirmed deaths, due to inadequate safety equipment and the shortage of trained staff and volunteers. Moreover, the government's social distancing guidelines did not allow large numbers of neighbours and relatives to attend the funeral (*Janazah*) prayer. The lockdown and social distancing also affected bereavement support for bereaved families, as people could not visit them to offer condolences and social support, which further saddened and devastated friends, relatives and loved ones of the deceased person.

Methodology

Due to my interest in the matters relating to urban inequalities, this study aimed to explore the challenges faced by the Bangladeshi Muslims in relation to funeral and mourning rituals at the community level while adhering to the social distancing rules. This study has ethnographic roots[5] because I am British-Bangladeshi and I have purposively chosen to live in London (England) and Edinburgh (Scotland). I have used my social connections with Bangladeshi people, and talked to three informants in London and one informant in Edinburgh. One of the informants is a woman (the widow of a COVID-19 victim), while the others are men. The informants provided funeral narratives of five COVID-19-related deaths and one non-COVID-19 death. All six deceased persons were Bangladeshi and were employed in public-facing jobs (that is, minicab driving, restaurant worker in Domino's Pizza, KFC and other food outlets) and had underlying health conditions. The deceased persons are all male, and they were the first people from their family/lineage to be buried in the UK regardless of any prior wish to be buried in Bangladesh via repatriation.

The interviews were conducted in Bengali over the phone in May 2020 after obtaining informed consent from the participants. The phone conversations were guided by a pre-developed checklist, and all informants and deceased are anonymised – the real names of the participants and deceased are masked with fictitious names The highest standards of ethical conduct were adhered to in line with the UK Social Research Association ethical guidelines and the General Data Protection Regulation (UK GDPR) in line with Data Protection Act 2018. The purpose of the study was communicated to participants, as well as their entitlement to withdraw from the research at any time until March 2021. Alongside analysis of this primary data, extensive secondary data analysis was carried out. Sources included reputable media reports, guidance by the government, the British Islamic Medical Association (BIMA, 2000) and the National Burial Council, previous and other research carried out over the same period. These sources of data helped to triangulate and add validity to the findings.

Findings

The study was conceptualised from an urban planning perspective with a view to exploring the state of (urban) inclusion of the Bangladeshi communities on the question of specific funeral and bereavement needs. The funeral experiences as reflected by the informants are discussed in the following sub-sections: dying in isolation with no spiritual support, waiting time to proceed the funeral rituals, regulations on washing and shrouding of the dead body, arranging the expensive funeral cost, socially distanced funeral prayer (*Janazah*) and socially distanced mourning.

Dying in isolation with no spiritual support (Gunaratnam, 2020)

The emotional turmoil of COVID-19 started with the pandemic reality of dying in isolation, separated from loved ones, with no spiritual end-of-life support. The physical and cognitive aspects of COVID-19 deaths exemplify a 'bad death', as people were dying with physical discomfort, breathing difficulty, social isolation and psychological distress

(Carr, Boerner and Moorman, 2020). Because of the highly contagious nature of the virus, hospitals and care homes prevented all visitors, including spiritual clerics, until the government vowed to give families the 'right to say goodbye' to loved ones from mid-April 2020. It was speculated that some critically-ill Bangladeshi patients might face difficulties in describing their illness because of language barriers, as they could not get the help of an interpreter or family member in the pandemic situation (Croxford, 2020; Islam and Netto, 2020).

Muslims believe that listening to the holy Quranic verses and pronouncing the auspicious words, the '*kalema*', reduce the pain of death. Therefore, spiritual end-of-life support is important for devoted Muslims (Yarrington, 2010; Maravia, 2020). The distress associated with a 'bad death' increased the anxiety and pain of the family and loved ones of dying persons affected by COVID-19 (Maddrell et al., 2018). One of the informants, Khatun (aged 39, the widow of a COVID-19-related deceased person, mother of four children) said that her husband (aged 49) was admitted to University College London Hospital in Euston, London for cancer treatment in mid-March 2020. After surgery, he developed COVID-19 symptoms and later tested COVID-19 positive. She said:

> I was frustrated and asked the hospital staff how the virus got into him while he was in intensive care ... I was devastated, the hospital sent me home and advised me to isolate myself with rest of the family ... In next few days, I called the hospital and begged them to visit visiting my husband but until the day before his death, they did not allow me to meet him. He died alone, no one there to read the Quran to ease his pain.

The need to extend spiritual support for those dying from COVID-19 in isolation also received public attention (Walker and Booth, 2020) and later end-of-life spiritual support was arranged for patients dying during the pandemic in an NHS setting.

My informant, Dr Zaman said:

> My neighbour's [Mr Amin, aged 55+, an Uber driver with an underlying health condition] family saw him before they removed the ventilator through a video call from the doctor. A religious cleric [*Maulana*] was there who recited the holy verses when life support was being removed.

Although in some cases, staff members in the hospital and care homes facilitated the last family conversation/time via phone or video conference call, not everyone was fortunate enough to say goodbye to their loved one during the pandemic and had to accept death in isolation.

Waiting time to procced the funeral rituals

In Islam, the deceased person should be buried as soon as possible, which is widely practised in Bangladesh.[6] In the UK, the burial process could not be officially started until the death certificate was obtained from a government registry office, which requires processing time to follow the various steps. During the lockdown restrictions, the family/friends of the deceased had to depend on emails/web-based correspondence (instead of physical visits) to process death certificates, which took more time than usual.

> My friends (Bangladeshis living in close proximity) helped me to get the death certificate, but the main interview was attended by me online. The procedure took longer than usual because we could not visit the office because of the lockdown. We had to wait 2–3 days for any email reply each time during the processing of the death certificate.
>
> (Khatun, 39)

After obtaining the death certificate, the family or friends could begin the funeral rituals by appointing a funeral director, who then collects the body from the hospital or home. During the lockdown, government offices had reduced their service, which elongated the processing time of death certificates and, therefore, contributed additional delays in staging the funeral and burial rites.

Regulations on washing and shrouding of the dead body

On 30 March 2020, the British Islamic Medical Association (BIMA)[7] and the National Burial Council[8] published guidance for handling suspected and confirmed COVID-19 deaths, with a detailed elaboration of *ghusl* practice (such as, wearing appropriate safety gear-PPE for *ghusl* performers, covering the mouth of the deceased person with a mask, and so on). Later, most funeral directories returned to funeral arrangements offering *ghusl*, while others offered *tayammum* (that is, dry washing) due to inadequate safety gear and the shortage of trained staff/volunteers (Maravia, 2020). Khatun's late husband did not have a *ghusl* before burial, instead he received *tayammum*: 'The funeral service did not wash my husband because of the possibility of disease transmission, but he got the *tayammum*, which is also fine due to the infectious circumstance.' In Bangladesh, *ghusl* is treated as an obligatory funeral ritual. My informants mentioned that some Asian-Muslims wanted to hide any evidence of the infection, because of fear of getting an improper funeral without *ghusl* and shrouding. Though some funeral services were offering *ghusl* and *tayammum* according to BIMA guidance, the satisfaction level varied, as one of my informants, Anis, said: 'Looking at my friend's face before the burial, I was in doubt whether he got the *ghusl*. The funeral service told us that they had performed the *ghusl* but no one from the family was allowed to see the *ghusl*.'

It should be noted that most funeral directories in London were overwhelmed by the high number of deaths and staff shortages when the pandemic had started to surface in the UK.

Expensive funeral costs

My informants reflected that the overhead costs inclusive of a burial plot or a layer ranged between £3,500 and £4,000. Where a family of the deceased could not afford the cost, the local Bangladeshi community arranged payments for the funeral. Moreover, one of the interviewees mentioned that a London-based funeral charity funded the funeral of a young Bangladeshi COVID-19 victim as his friends were unable to pay for the funeral (Bakar, 2020). My informant, Anowar, who lives in Edinburgh, mentioned that a late friend (who died during the pandemic) used to send most of his earnings back home to support his family, and so he did not have savings of thousand of pounds that could be used for his funeral expenses:

> The coffin costs £700, funeral is expensive. Government reimburse £1,200 to contribute to the funeral cost for the people who receive benefit. But the people who don't receive benefit, they have to arrange their[own] funeral cost. My friend (who died from a non-COVID-19 cause) was not a benefit recipient as he was a chef in a restaurant. He did not have any family here and so his Bangladeshi friends in Edinburgh paid the expense.

Most of my informants heard that there is a council scheme to reimburse some of the funeral costs for poorer people However, the scheme did not help Bangladeshi people during the pandemic and they relied on family/community initiatives or charity to finance the funeral cost.

*Socially distanced funeral prayer (*Janazah*)*

The funeral prayer is performed in congregation and is one of the important rites for the soul's wellbeing in the Islamic belief. A Muslim presence at the *Janazah* prayer is considered to be beneficial to seek pardon for the deceased.[9] However, the pandemic limited the number of people attending the *Janazah*; in some cases it was limited to five people. It was devastating for some who could not, in order to adhere to social distancing rules, attend the *Janazah* of their late friends or family members. My informant, Anis, wanted to attend the *Janazah* of his late friend as they had prayed together in the mosque for the last five years. On the day of the funeral, he went to the funeral home knowing that he could not attend *Janazah* because the five *Janazah*-participants were selected beforehand and he was not enlisted. Fortunately, the funeral director allowed him to pay his last tribute to his friend through attending the *Janazah* prayer:

> I parked the car in the premise [of the funeral home]. One of their staff asked me if I came to attend the *Janazah*. I did not answer as I knew I was not enlisted to attend the *Janazah*. However, they allowed me to attend the *Janazah* as the sixth attendee.

The male[10] informants who attended the *Janazah* prayer during the pandemic mentioned that funeral directors decided the number of people who could attend. In Edinburgh, the Scottish Muslim Funeral Services[11] ruled out allowing ten people. Anowar, considering the Scottish Muslim Funeral Services ruling, arranged *janazah* prayers in the graveyard, and they allowed as many as 16 (or more) people, as long as social distancing measures were ensured.

During the pandemic, video conferencing allowed some people to virtually attend the funeral of their loved ones.

I asked the informants whether Bangladeshi people used video conferencing aids to virtually attend the funeral. One of my informants, Anis, said video conferencing and photography were forbidden by the funeral directory. Two other informants said the funeral directory allowed them to take photographs or make a video conference call to connect with loved ones. In Edinburgh, the family members of the Bangladeshi man (non-COVID-19 death) attended the funeral via a video conference call from Bangladesh. My informant, Anowar, reflected:

> I made the video call to Bangladesh so that his family (wife and daughters) can see his face for the last time. The girls were crying a lot and the environment was saddened by the situation. The poor girls didn't even see their father's face properly as most part of his face was covered by a surgical mask[12] for safety reason.

By and large, people who died during lockdown restrictions received a *Janazah* prayer, although family members and friends could not in some cases attend. Attending funerals through video conference calls did not ease the grief of the mourners; however, it helped some family members to pay their respects virtually – especially those whose families were living overseas and their desire for repatriation of the body could not be arranged due to international travel restrictions.

Socially distanced mourning

The Islamic mourning practices include frequent visits to the bereaved family to offer condolences and other support (for example, providing food). The COVID-19 crisis restricted the ways in which bereavement support could be offered; therefore, neighbours and relatives were in distress as they could not emotionally support the bereaved family in person. My informant Dr Zaman said his neighbour's (Amin, who was an Uber driver with an underlying health condition) wife did not want to disclose her husband's cause of death (COVID-19) in public because she feared that people might label their family unclean – which symbolises the fear of stigmatisation of blaming immigrant groups for the spread of dangerous pathogens (Markel and Stern, 2002). Dr Zaman said:

> My neighbour [the deceased] was a social person, he had many friends and there were gatherings in his house every now and then. Now, no one could visit his family to offer condolences. His friends leave the food at doorsteps and call them to take it. It's quite sad but we all have to accept it.

The informants reflected the Bangladeshi community as a whole was supporting people in distress; however, the lockdown and social distancing rules hampered the usual bereavement practices and the bereaved family remained excluded from the condolences and comfort they deserved. This unprecedented situation demands more community connection and government support to acknowledge the challenges from this pandemic surge.

Recommendations for future practice

All informants suggested that the volume of the available funeral services (for example, the number of burial plots and funeral directories) needs to be increased to fulfil specific funeral rituals (for example, quick burial) in other unprecedented situations in the future. There is a need to train more volunteers to perform the *ghusl*, using safety equipment if necessary. Also, the current population growth trend suggests that the Muslim population is increasing in both London and Edinburgh, so there is a need for more burial plots and funeral services to meet the needs of these communities in the future. Moreover, more planning and policy interventions are needed in post-industrial conurbations for wider inclusion of the British-Bangladeshi people in UK society by ensuring their funeral needs are met.

Moreover, the COVID-19 situation has changed the view of some British-Bangladeshi people in terms of where they want to be buried. People who initially thought to be buried in Bangladesh through repatriation have seemingly changed their minds, and want to be to be buried in London. My informant, Anis (who immigrated from Italy a few years ago) was contributing to a community-based insurance scheme for repatriation when he was living in Italy; now he no longer wants to be buried in Bangladesh.

> I have visited the Muslim cemetery in Ilford [the Garden of Peace]. It is a peaceful place. I wish to be buried there if I die in London. I was contributing in an insurance scheme for repatriation when I was in Italy because the Muslim funeral service was not convenient there. In London, Muslims are satisfied with the funeral services and they want to be buried here instead of repatriation.

Almost all informants mentioned they had joined community-led insurance schemes that enable the community to pay off the funeral expenses of the participants after their death. The interviewees reflected that British-Bangladeshis with an immigration history seldom think about dying rather than thriving in a foreign land:

> Bangladeshis do not want to discuss the topic related to 'death', either they fear or they feel uncomfortable to have a conservation on death. There needs to be more talk within and beyond the Bangladeshi community on funeral needs and challenges based on the learning from the pandemic.
> (Anowar)

Most of the respondents reflected that there needs to be more support from local councils and government for the bereaved family. There was no planning in place to tackle the higher number of funerals and bereavement needs, even though the news/media had sufficiently covered the outbreak and emerging disease threats of the novel coronavirus (SARS-CoV-2) because of uncontrolled international mobility (Sun et al, 2011). All ethnic and religious communities and local and regional governments need to devise innovative ways to face the unprecedented challenges. My informant, Dr Zaman, reflected: 'The systems had failed worldwide. Bill Gates[13] predicted today's situation in 2015, but biologist, epidemiologist, virologist failed to predict the novel Coronavirus outbreak. We could have prepared and eradicated it. We need to use science in more practical and meaningful ways.' Nevertheless, Anowar mentioned there were graves of Scottish people in Sylhet who were buried in Bangladesh from the seventeenth to the twentieth centuries:[14]

> Some Scottish people are resting in peace in Bangladesh who died hundred years ago. My friend is resting in peace in Scotland. History repeats. I wish our [Bangladeshi Muslims'] graves could be identified after hundred years like the graves of the Scottish people were identified by the British people [that is, identified by British Association for Cemeteries in South Asia-BACSA].

The COVID-19 pandemic not only affected the Bangladeshi community with an unequal impact, but also highlighted other sociocultural needs that require attention for wider inclusion of the ethnic minority communities in the UK.

Conclusion

Death is not only an individual experience but invites a string of multifaceted events with social, religious, cultural, and spiritual connotations at community level. The needs associated with the funeral rites of ethnic minority groups are less discussed in the academic literature. However, the pandemic has illustrated the importance of discursive dialogues involving the public, policy makers, council officials, planners, scientists, public health experts and academics for wider inclusion of British-Bangladeshi communities. The challenges posed by the pandemic need to be treated with great importance so that expert-led and better planning interventions can be applied to meet the funeral and bereavement needs of Bangladeshi people in future.

Notes

[1] Key workers are the people whose jobs are vital to public health and safety during the coronavirus lockdown. Key workers include those working in health and social care, education, utilities and communication, food and necessary goods, transport, key public services, national and local governments: see https://www.ons.gov.uk/employmentandlabourmarket/peopleinwork/earningsandworkinghours/articles/coronavirusandkeyworkersintheuk/2020-05-15.

[2] Author's ethnographic observation.

[3] 'Myth of return' indicates a yearning to be buried in Bangladesh, but does not necessarily mean returning to Bangladesh when alive.

[4] Al-Tirmidhi, 1998, Hadith No. 998: https://hamariweb.com/islam/hadith/jami-at-tirmidhi-998/

[5] 'Ethnography and participant observation entail the extended involvement of the researcher in the social life of those he or she studied' (Creswell, 2013: 431).

[6] Author's ethnographic observation suggest that except unnatural death (for example, deaths from road accidents, suicide, murder and so on, when an autopsy is mandatory), burial is quick and does not depend upon obtaining a death certificate.

[7] https://mcb.org.uk/community/COVID-19-muslim-burial-resources/

[8] https://eternalgardens.org.uk/wp-content/uploads/2020/04/NBC-Summary-Guidance-NO.3-for-BURIAL-of-COVID-19-death-7-April.pdf

[9] https://muflihun.com/muslim/4/2072

[10] Only males are supposed to attend the Janazah according to Sunni Islam (Yarrington, 2010).

[11] The only Muslim funeral directory in Edinburgh.

[12] The National Burial Council suggested that the mouth of the deceased person should be covered with a mask; see https://eternalgardens.org.uk/wp-content/uploads/2020/04/NBC-Summary-Guidance-NO.3-for-BURIAL-of-COVID-19-death-7-April.pdf

[13] https://www.youtube.com/watch?v=6Af6b_wyiwI

[14] The book *Tombs in Tea: Tea Garden Cemeteries, Sylhet, Bangladesh* (BACSA, 2001: 82) identified 20 graves belonging to deceased Scots.

References

Afiouni, N. (2019) 'Transformations of the burial places of Muslims in Greater London', *Review of the Muslim Worlds and of the Mediterranean*, 146(2): 139–154. doi: 10.4000/remmm.13769

Bakar, F. (2020) 'Meet the man arranging Muslim funerals for those in need in the coronavirus pandemic', Metro, 24 April [online]. Available from: https://metro.co.uk/2020/04/24/man-dealing-coronavirus-burial-poverty-12588160/

Carr, D., Boerner, K. and Moorman, S. (2020) 'Bereavement in the time of coronavirus: unprecedented challenges demand novel interventions', *Journal of Aging and Social Policy*, 32(4–5), 425–431. doi: 10.1080/08959420.2020.1764320.

Cheraghi, M.A., Payne, S. and Salsali, M. (2005) 'Spiritual aspects of end-of-life care for Muslim patients: experiences from Iran', *International Journal of Palliative Nursing*, 11(9): 468–474. doi: 10.12968/ijpn.2005.11.9.19781

Creswell, J.W. (2013) *Qualitative Inquiry and Research Design: Choosing Among Five Approaches*, US: SAGE.

Croxford, R. (2020) 'Coronavirus: ethnic minorities "are a third" of patients', *BBC News*, 12 April. doi: 10.1080/08959420.2020.1764320

Gardner, K. (1998) 'Death, burial and bereavement amongst Bengali Muslims in Tower Hamlets, East London', *Journal of Ethnic and Migration Studies*, 24(3): 507–521. doi: 10.1080/1369183X.1998.9976647

Gunaratnam, Y. (2000) 'People who need end-of-life care shouldn't have to die alone because of coronavirus', *The Guardian*, 17 April [online]. Available from: https://www.theguardian.com/society/2020/apr/17/people-who-need-end-of-life-care-shouldnt-have-to-die-alone-because-of-coronavirus

Hadith, The (p 948, Sahih Muslim, Book of Prayers, Vol. 2, Hadith 2072). Available from: https://muflihun.com/ muslim/4/2072

Hunter, A. (2016) 'Deathscapes in diaspora: contesting space and negotiating home in contexts of post-migration diversity', *Social and Cultural Geography*, 17(2): 247–261. doi: 10.1080/14649365.2015.1059472

Islam, F. (2019) 'The impact of Olympic-led urban regeneration on ethnic minority residents in London: a right to the city perspective', PhD thesis, Heriot-Watt University.

Islam, F. and Netto, G. (2020) ' "The virus does not discriminate": debunking the myth: the unequal impact of COVID-19 on ethnic minority groups', *Radical Statistics Journal*, 126: 19– 23 [Online]. Available from: https://www.radstats.org.uk/journal/issue126/

Jahangir, M.S. and Hamid, W. (2020) 'Mapping mourning among Muslims of Kashmir: analysis of religious principles and current practices', *Sage Journals*. doi: 10.1177/0030222820911544

Maddrell, A. (2016) 'Cartographier le chagrin. Cadre conceptuel pour comprendre les dimensions spatiales de la perte, du deuil et du souvenir', *Social and Cultural Geography*, 17(2): 166–188. doi : 10.1080/14649365.2015.1075579

Maddrell, A, Beebeejaun, Y., McClymont, K., McNally, D., Mathijssen, B. and Abid Dogra, S. (2018) 'Deathscapes and diversity in England and Wales: setting an agenda', *Revista d'Etnologia de Catalunya*, 43: 38–53.

Maravia, U. (2020) 'Rationale for suspending Friday prayers, funerary rites, and fasting Ramadan during COVID-19: an analysis of the fatawa related to the coronavirus', *Journal of the British Islamic Medical Association*, 4(2): 1–6.

Markel, H. and Stern, A.M. (2002) 'The foreignness of germs: the persistent association of immigrants and disease in American society', *Milbank Quarterly*, 80(4): 757–788. doi: 10.1111/1468-0009.00030

Office for National Statistics (2011) 'CT0575 2011 Census - ethnic group (write-in response) by religion – England', ONS [online]. Available from: https://www.ons.gov.uk/peoplepopulationandcommunity/culturalidentity/ethnicity/adhocs/005528ct05752011censusethnicgroupwriteinresponsebyreligionengland

Parveen, N. (2020) 'The Muslims bereaved cruelly deprived of closure by coronavirus', *The Guardian*, 7 June [online]. Available from: https://www.theguardian.com/world/2020/jul/07/the-muslim-bereaved-cruelly-deprived-of-closure-by-coronavirus

Public Health England (PHE) (2020a) 'Disparities in the risk and outcomes from COVID-19', *Gov.uk* [online]. Available from: https://assets.publishing.service.gov.uk/government/uploads/system/uploads/attachment_data/file/892085/disparities_review.pdf

—— (2020b) 'Beyond the data: understanding the impact of COVID-19 on BAME groups', *Gov.uk* [online]. Available from: https://assets.publishing.service.gov.uk/government/uploads/system/uploads/attachment_data/file/892376/COVID_stakeholder_engagement_synthesis_beyond_the_data.pdf

Radford, J.A. and Farrington, S.M. (2001) *Tombs in Tea: Tea garden Cemeteries*. Sylhet, Bangladesh: BACSA (British Association for Cemeteries in South Asia).

Reza, M.M. (2020) 'Rites de passage in Bangladesh: Nilphamari perspective', *Journal of ELT and Education*, 3(01–02): 1–7.

Stevenson, O., Kenten, C. and Maddrell, A. (2016) 'Et maintenant la fin approche: revitaliser et politiser les géographies du trépas, de la mort et du deuil', *Social and Cultural Geography*, 17(2): 153–165. doi: 10.1080/14649365.2016.1152396.

Sun, C., Yang, W., Arino, J. and Khan, K. (2011) 'Effect of media-induced social distancing on disease transmission in a two patch setting', *Mathematical Biosciences*, 230(2): 87–95. doi: 10.1016/j.mbs.2011.01.005

Walker, P. and Booth, R. (2020) 'Hancock vows to give families "right to say goodbye" to loved ones', *The Guardian*, 15 April [online]. Available from: https://www.theguardian.com/world/2020/apr/15/families-to-be-allowed-to-say-goodbye-to-dying-relatives-in-care-homes

Watt, P. (2008) 'The only class in town? Gentrification and the middle-class colonization of the city and the urban imagination', *International Journal of Urban and Regional Research*, 32(1): 206–211. doi: 10.1111/j.1468-2427.2008.00769.x

Yarrington, M.D. (2010) 'Lived Islam in Bangladesh: contemporary religious discourse between Ahl-i- Hadith, "Hanafis" and authoritative texts, with special reference to al-barzakh', PhD thesis, University of Edinburgh.

EIGHT

Racial justice and equalities law: progress, pandemic and potential

Robin Richardson

Introduction

The landmark act of parliament known as the Equality Act 2010 received royal assent on 8 April 2010 and came into effect a few months later, on 1 October. It was the culmination of a legislative process that, by 2010, had lasted in the UK for at least 45 years, had been deeply influenced by parallel developments in other European countries and the US, and had entailed much campaigning and deliberating, and much organising and reorganising (Hepple, 2010). Its most promising features included (1) a general duty imposed on all public authorities not only to avoid adverse impacts of their policies and practices but also to promote greater equality of outcome, (2) specific duties whose purpose was to support, focus and clarify the general duty and (3) a holistic approach to non-discrimination, namely one that was based on the commonalities between different strands and facets of diversity such as age, disability, gender, race, religion and sexuality.

One significant and indeed foundational piece of reorganising occurred in the UK in 2007. During the last week of September that year, farewell newsletters were sent to their friends, contacts and supporters by the Equal Opportunities Commission (EOC, founded in 1975), the Commission for Racial Equality (CRE, founded in 1976) and the Disability Rights Commission (DRC, founded in 1999). All three of these had been supporting an aspect of equalities legislation in England, Scotland and Wales. A few days later, on 28 September, all three would cease to exist as separate entities, and from 1 October 2007 onwards each would instead be part of a new body formed by each merging with the other two. The CRE told its friends it was becoming part of a body to be named the CEHR, the Commission for Equality and Human Rights. The DRC and the EOC, however, each made a slightly different announcement. They for their part, they said, were joining a body to be named as the EHRC, the Equality and Human Rights Commission.

At the time, the confusion did not appear to matter. Certainly it was trivial compared with other issues facing the fields of disability, gender and race equality at that time. Nevertheless, the confusion looked suspicious and ominous. If the three founding partners in the new equalities commission could not agree on its very name, what were the chances they could work together harmoniously, let alone with synergy, in the months and years ahead?

There were further anxieties too. What were the chances the new commission would in due course welcome and integrate new legal concerns around age, religion and sexual orientation, and – as a matter of urgency – weave equalities and human rights into a seamless web of thinking and action? Would it be capable of creating and maintaining a holistic and intersectional approach to equality, and fit-for-purpose systems of leadership, responsibility and day-to-day administration? Would it realise, in both senses of this word (be aware of, make real), its potential? Would it truly be able effectively to challenge public bodies in England, Scotland and Wales to have due regard for equality in their mainstream planning, procedures and activities, and assertively and effectively speak truth to power? A particularly relevant question in the light of what occurred some ten years later, and in the context of this book, would the new commission speak and act holistically with robust clarity if and when there was a global crisis? For example, if there were a pandemic or syndemic (Singer, 2009) arising from a perfect storm of intersecting causes, and leading to a tempest of mutually reinforcing inequalities and unfairness? Not least, how if at all, would the new commission have due regard for the wider context – political, socioeconomic, cultural – in which it would necessarily be operating, and how would such regard be manifest in the commission's relationships with central government? Time would tell.

In the event, as outlined in this chapter, the Equality Act did not achieve its potential. This was primarily because successive governments from 2010 onwards were lukewarm, at best, in support for it. Also, however, equality organisations and lobbies did not forge cooperative ways of working together and supporting each other, and were, in consequence, unable effectively to speak truth to power. How this happened will hopefully be explored, centrally or at least incidentally and in the margins, by the UK COVID-19 Inquiry (Cabinet Office, 2022).

Review of the decade, 2010–2020

Shortly after the Equalities Bill received royal assent as the Equality Act 2010 there was a general election, followed by a new administration, the coalition of Conservatives and Liberal Democrats led by David Cameron. Initially the outlook for equalities was promising. Barely five weeks after the election (9 June 2010) the new Home Secretary and Minister for Women and Equalities (Theresa May) wrote formally to cabinet colleagues to remind them of their legal duty to have due regard for equality in relation to disability, ethnicity and gender (Dodd, 2010). She also reminded them of forthcoming duties in relation to age, religion, sexual orientation and transgender rights. Her immediate concern was the likely impact on equalities from imminent budgetary cuts. Her letter was also relevant, however, for a full range of government policies, actions and decisions. She warned that 'there are real risks that women, ethnic minorities, disabled people and older people will be disproportionately affected' by the cuts. All four of these groups, she pointed out, use public services more than the population as a whole, and the majority of people in receipt of tax credits and welfare payments belonged to these groups. And all four, incidentally but significantly, would be prominent among those most negatively impacted in due course by COVID-19 (Public Health England, 2020; Younge, 2021).

May's letter to cabinet colleagues was presumably drafted by senior civil servants at the Home Office who had until recently been closely involved in preparations for the Equality Act, and who were in consequence thoroughly familiar with the Act's intentions and potential. These were not, however, the only people who had access to the Home Secretary and who were keen to influence her. Also, there were special advisers ('spads') who had close links with the Conservative party and with right-wing thinktanks, opinion leaders, magazines and newspapers. (Discussions prior or subsequent to 2010 included Palmer, 1986; Murray, 2006; Scruton, 2014.) Theresa May not only commended the Equality Act to her cabinet colleagues but also began to preside over a series of measures and regulations whose avowed purpose was to maintain a 'hostile environment' for undocumented refugees and asylum-seekers, and whose effect was also to instill anxiety and insecurity among people who were citizens or residents of long standing, but felt alien and vulnerable as a consequence of their actual or perceived cultural, ethnic, racial or religious identity (Liberty, 2019).

Critical opposition to the Equality Act was clearly reflected in a speech that the Home Secretary delivered at a community centre in south London on 17 November 2010 (May, 2010) At one point in this speech, May referred to section 1 of the Act, and to the requirement that public bodies should exercise their functions 'in a way that is designed to reduce the inequalities of outcome which result from socio-economic disadvantage'. The Act had come into force on 1 October 2010, but section 1 had not yet been formally activated. May announced that section 1 would not be activated, enacted or commenced. She did not, however, use the legal terms 'activated', 'enacted' and 'commenced', but reportedly said the duty would be 'ditched' (Slack, 2010) or 'scrapped' (the term that appeared in the text of her speech as published). Nor, apparently, did May refrain from political point-scoring, sarcasm, misrepresentation and caricature. 'Just look', she said, 'at the socio-economic duty which Harriet Harman [the senior Labour politician who had steered the Bill through to its conclusion] slipped into the Equality Act at the last minute'. Many, she added, 'have called it socialism in one clause … Harman's Law, as it affectionately came to be known, meant to force public authorities to take into account disadvantage and inequalities when making decisions about their policies'.

In reality, May continued, the socioeconomic duty would have been 'just another bureaucratic box to be ticked'. The Labour party, she said, 'thought they could make things better by simply passing a law saying that they should be made better. That was as ridiculous as it was simplistic and that is why we are announcing that we are scrapping Harman's Law for good' (Slack, 2010). The phrase 'socialism in one clause' had been used by a member of the Labour cabinet in early 2009 when commenting on and commending a white paper on social mobility. A columnist on *The Guardian* had reported:

> The government will create a new over-arching law creating a duty on the whole public sector to narrow the gap between the rich and the poor. This single legal duty will stand as the main frame from which all other

equality legislation flows. Race, gender and disability injustices are all subsets of the one great inequality – class. It trumps them all. The gap between rich and poor in Britain is greater than in almost all rich nations, putting the UK with the United States among the most unequal.
(Toynbee, 2009)

It was, perhaps, not surprising, though certainly it was disappointing and most unfortunate, that the proposed socioeconomic duty was not probed, debated and clarified in the closing stages of the Bill's committee stage in the House of Commons. If it had been, the COVID-19 pandemic that hit the UK from 2019–2020 onwards might have been handled with much greater sensitivity and effectiveness, less hospitalisation and intensive care support and fewer deaths, and far fewer disparities in the outcomes for different groups and communities. For example, there might have been much more attention to what public health professionals call 'the social determinants of health' (Marmot, 2009; APPG for Longevity, 2020) – the pathology not only of the individual human body but also of wider society. As it was, the nearest the socioeconomic duty got to parliamentary scrutiny in 2009–2010 was in a brief debate in the House of Lords on the day following the Home Secretary's speech at a community centre. Speakers from both parties in the coalition government claimed that the duty was unenforceable and that was why it was not going to be enacted. The response of the Opposition spokesperson (Baroness Royall of Blaisdon) was scathing, but calm and clear:

> The socio-economic clause in the Equalities [sic] Act is a far cry from socialism in one clause, as the Home Secretary seeks to characterise it. It is a measure aimed simply at getting public organisations to think about the impact of their decisions on people who are disadvantaged. Many of these organisations already do

so, and this mean-minded little announcement will in all probability not change that ... Despite the Home Secretary's claims that the Government are all about fairness, is it not the case that the Government do not believe that they have any responsibility to deliver a fairer society?

(Royall, 2010)

With regard to the government's claim that the socioeconomic duty could not be enforced, and therefore should be 'scrapped', the Opposition spokesperson in the House of Lords did not make the obvious point that conceptual and procedural matters relating to the duty could readily be modelled on those that were already in force in relation to the public sector equality duty (PSED) required by section 149 of the Act. Namely, there would be a general duty of due regard complemented and focused by specific duties to publish (1) information and (2) measurable objectives.

In relation to public health, a socioeconomic duty stressing due regard for fairness (as summarised in, among many other places, Marmot 2020; Razai et al 2020a, 2020b; Bambra et al, 2021; Cooper and Szreter, 2021; Horton 2021; Race Disparity Unit, 2021) would have referred to data relating to life expectation, chronic illness and morbidity, and mental health and wellbeing at various ages and stages throughout a person's life.

In countries throughout the world, and at all times in history, the incidence of health and illness follows a social gradient: the lower a person's socioeconomic situation, the worse their health and the lower their life expectation is likely to be, as also their expectation of a healthy old age. In addition, decades of research show that adverse childhood experiences (ACEs) – for example abuse, neglect, trauma, domestic conflict and violence, low income, racism and hostile environments – can have detrimental impacts on a person's long-term physical and mental health, leading in due course to accelerated ageing, chronic disease, disability and premature death (Villines, 2020; Wu, 2020). Experiences of stress and adversity in childhood may also influence a person's genes and therefore be passed on to future generations (Marmot et al, 2021). In addition, they include high-risk occupations, for example those that entail close interaction with members of the general public. Although separate for the sake of making a list, social determinants of health frequently interact with each other and are mutually reinforcing – often, it is said, they may be 'causes of causes'. The shorthand generic term for them, socioeconomic, is not ideal. But it is widely known and used, and is prominent in the Equality Act 2010, though as mentioned here earlier, not yet 'commenced' or 'activated' (the technical legal words) in English law. The term is, however, enshrined in Scottish and Welsh law, and in the regulations and requirements of a handful of English local authorities. It would, therefore, be relevant and valuable, particularly in the light of the disparities and inequities highlighted by the COVID-19 pandemic, to reopen debate and deliberation about it. Socioeconomic circumstances would not be a protected characteristic in equalities law, but would be explicitly seen as the context in which unfair discrimination and unequal equal opportunities may occur and, therefore, for which there would need to be due regard. They are appropriately measured with reference to the index of multiple deprivation (IMD), not to a single factor such as low household income or (in the education system) eligibility for free school meals (Pickett, 2021).

Similar to the concept of IMD is LBN (left-behind neighbourhood). The concept of LBNs also has the practical advantage of being acceptable across a wide political spectrum, as attested by the existence of a vigorous all-party parliamentary group (APPG) at Westminster. There is full information in a report by Munford and Mott et al, 2022, and in an academic briefing paper by Darlington-Pollock et al, 2021. Munford and Mott (2022) note that a woman born in an LBN can expect to have 57.3 healthy years on average, compared with 64.8 healthy years nationally, and that a man born in an LBN can expect to have 55.9 healthy years on average, compared with 63.5 years nationally. They note also that LBNs have a higher proportion of people who self-report their health to be bad or very bad than in England as a whole. Of the 225 LBNs, 223 have higher levels of bad or very bad health than the national average, and a higher prevalence of 15 of the most common 21 health conditions compared with England as a whole, including high blood pressure, obesity and chronic lung conditions (Munford et al, 2022). In addition, people in LBNs claim almost double the amount of incapacity benefits due to mental health related conditions. It is as a result of these health disparities that people in LBNs are living shorter lives than elsewhere, with around 7.5 fewer years' life in good health. All 225 LBNs have lower healthy life expectancy than the national average for females and males, and life expectancy for those living in LBNs actually decreased in the mid-2010s. Further, people living in LBNs are 46 per cent more likely to die of COVID-19 compared with the national average. (All these statistics are reported by Munford and Mott, 2022: 8–13.) Other research has shown that only 9 per cent of white British people live in the most deprived tenth of neighbourhoods in England, compared with 31 per cent of people of Pakistani heritage, 19 per cent of Bangladeshi, and 15 per cent of Caribbean and African.

Tackling these health disparities, Munford and Mott point out, will not only improve the lives of millions of citizens, but will also bring significant savings to the taxpayer:

> If the health outcomes in local authorities that contain LBNs were brought up to the same level as in the rest of the country, an extra £29.8bn could be put into the country's economy. Where local residents have the right capacity and support in place, there is significant potential for communities to develop effective, locally appropriate and preventative solutions, with huge potential benefits for an over-stretched health service.

The concept of LBN, then, has much promising potential. Other signs of promise and hope include recent developments in Scotland and Wales, and in certain English towns and cities. It was not widely appreciated in 2010 that the Home Secretary had the power to 'ditch' or 'scrap' (her words) section 1 of the Act in England, but not in the devolved administrations of Scotland or Wales. In due course, accordingly, section 1 was commenced in both these jurisdictions.

The Fairer Scotland Duty, Part 1 of the Equality Act 2010, came into force in Scotland from April 2018. It places a legal responsibility on certain public bodies in Scotland to actively consider ('pay due regard' to) how they can reduce inequalities of outcome caused by socioeconomic disadvantage, when making strategic decisions. The Scottish Government sees the new duty as 'an opportunity to do things differently and to put tackling inequality genuinely at the heart of key decision-making'. People in Scotland still experience, it notes, significant socioeconomic disadvantage and resulting inequalities of outcome. Over a million Scots are living in poverty, for example, including one in four children; and health inequalities and educational attainment gaps are wide (Scottish Government, 2018). And in Wales, since April 2021, public authorities are similarly required to have due regard for the need to develop scrutiny frameworks and conduct impact assessments on socioeconomic issues (Welsh Government, 2021).

All public bodies in the UK are already expected to formally and explicitly decide to affirm or reaffirm that they have due regard for the three needs named in the general duty ('the public sector equality duty') in the Equality Act 2010 and to observe the two specific duties (to provide information and to set objectives) that are intended to focus and support the general duty. They may also choose to revisit, revise and improve the guidance on these duties which the government issued shortly after 2010, but for the most part subsequently withdrew or itself disregarded (Richardson, 2022). Every public body can, in addition, choose to observe the socioeconomic duty in section 1 of the Equality Act 2010. Following a review of the local effects of COVID-19 (Mamluck and Jones, 2020), Bristol City Council made the following declaration:

> As well as looking at our statutory duties, as set out under the Public Sector Equality Duty, our strategy will also consider wider aspirations, such as reducing inequalities of outcome which result from socio-economic disadvantage. As part of our annual reporting of equalities and inclusion we will identify socio-economic trends and where we can focus our future efforts to reduce socio-economic inequalities.
>
> (Bristol City Council, 2021)

Equality organisations, including the Equality and Human Rights Commission, can develop and provide resources, consultancies and training events that will support implementation of the Equality Act's general and specific duties, and of the socioeconomic duty if so requested. (See also Liverpool City Region, 2021.)

Culture wars

Throughout the decade beginning in 2010 various thinktanks, politicians and opinion leaders in the US and UK spoke and wrote, and sometimes managed to legislate against, Critical Race Theory, unconscious bias training, affirmative action, decolonisation in the curricula of schools and universities, and concepts of white privilege and institutional and structural racism, defined as 'the processes of racism that are embedded in laws (local, state, and federal), policies, and practices of society and its institutions that provide advantages to ethnic groups deemed as superior, while differentially oppressing, disadvantaging, or otherwise neglecting ethnic groups viewed as inferior' (Razai et al, 2021a: 2). Sometimes, opposition to the concept of structural racism is expressed entirely openly and explicitly; sometimes, though, it uses dog-whistles and various codewords, for example 'woke' or 'wokery' and 'political correctness'. In effect, such criticisms favour and promote a hostile environment, not only towards those who are deemed to be 'others', but also towards academics, teachers, organisations and newspapers who are considered to be malign and destructive in their influence (Webber, 2022).

The tone and trend in such attacks on equalities legislation were strikingly evident in a speech given by Liz Truss, the Minister for Women and Equalities, in December 2020. It was reminiscent of the speech made by Theresa May almost exactly ten years previously, quoted here earlier. The text of the speech was redacted when printed on a government website and did not contain the words quoted here:

> As a comprehensive school student in Leeds in the 1980s, I was struck by the lip service that was paid to equality by the City Council while children from disadvantaged backgrounds were let down. While we were taught about racism and sexism, there was too little time spent making sure everyone could read and write. These ideas have their roots in post-modernist philosophy – pioneered by Foucault – that put societal power structures and labels ahead of individuals and their endeavours. In this school of thought, there is no space for evidence, as there is no objective view – truth and morality are all relative. Rather than promote policies that would have been a game-changer for the disenfranchised, like better education and business opportunities, there was a preference for symbolic gestures.
>
> (quoted in Meaden, 2020; Tolhurst, 2020)

Regarding lived experiences of oppression, and empathy and imaginative compassion towards the victims of oppression, there were two particularly dramatic, iconic, visceral and symbolic events in the summer of 2020 that may appropriately be recalled here as this chapter draws towards its close. One evoked present realities, the other evoked cruelties and structural violence in the past. Present realities were symbolised by the murder in Minneapolis of George Perry Floyd on 25 May. History was made vivid by the sight a fortnight later (7 June) of the statue of an infamous slave-trader, Edward Colston, being dumped into Bristol harbour. Each of these symbolic events on its own, but also the pair in juxtaposition with each other, galvanised and reinforced public anger, energy, resolution and hope throughout the world.

The story of non-discrimination law in the UK began with race relations legislation in 1965 and 1968. It is fitting, therefore, that the story should pause now with a further reminder from the racial justice field that marginalised, othered and oppressed lives matter. That said, in the overall task of developing a holistic view of equality, there is clearly still much to be done, still much unfinished business.

Conclusion

The Equality Act 2010 in the UK marked the culmination of 45 years of deliberation, campaigning and legislating, and had the clear potential to protect members of certain groups, backgrounds and communities from unfair discrimination in employment and the provision of services. In the years following 2010, however, the COVID-19 pandemic had a disproportionately negative impact on people with protected characteristics, as defined by the Act. It follows that the Act needs to be revisited, revised and re-emphasised. Among other measures, but crucially, this will involve (1) activating the Act's socioeconomic duty, (2) attending to needs and priorities in left-behind neighbourhoods (LBNs), and (3) addressing forms of inequality that are systemic and structural. Further, it is essential that equality organisations and lobbies should work more cooperatively with each other than hitherto, and that mutual support and learning among them should be encouraged and resourced by public bodies. The essential task is not only to 'build back better', as is often said, but also to build back fairer. If the new normal is not significantly fairer in its outcomes than the old, it will not be better. Arundhati Roy declares:

> Historically, pandemics have forced humans to break with the past and imagine their world anew. This one is no different. It is a portal, a gateway between one world and the next. We can choose to walk through it, dragging the carcasses of our prejudice and hatred, our avarice, our data banks and dead ideas. Or we can walk through lightly, with little luggage, ready to imagine another world. And ready to fight for it.
>
> (Roy, 2020)

References

All-Party Parliamentary Group for Longevity (2020) *The Health of the Nation*, London: APPG for Longevity and Longevity UK.

Bambra, C. et al (2021) *The Unequal Pandemic: COVID-19 and Health Inequalities*, Bristol: Policy Press.

Bristol City Council (2018, revised 2021) *Equality and Inclusion: Policy and Strategy, 2018–2023*, Bristol: Bristol City Council.

Cabinet Office (2022) 'UK COVID-19 Inquiry', Gov.uk [online]. Available from: https://www.gov.uk/government/publications/uk-covid-19-inquiry-terms-of-reference/uk-covid-19-inquiry-terms-of-reference

Cooper, H. and Szreter, S. (2021) *After the Virus: Lessons from the Past for a Better Future*, Cambridge: Cambridge University Press.

Darlington-Pollock, F. et al (2021) 'Briefing: what do "left behind" areas look like over time?', *Left Behind Neighbourhoods* [online]. Available from: https://www.appg-leftbehindneighbourhoods.org.uk/wp-content/uploads/2021/08/GDSL-Liverpool-University-Briefing.pdf

Dodd, V. (2010) 'Budget cuts could break equality laws, Theresa May warned chancellor', *The Guardian*, 3 August [online]. Available from: https://www.theguardian.com/politics/2010/aug/03/budget-cuts-equality-theresa-may

Equality Act (2010). 'Equality Act 2010', Legislation.gov.uk [online]. Available from: https://www.legislation.gov.uk/ukpga/2010/15/contents

Hepple, B. (2010) 'The new single Equality Act in Britain', *Equality Rights Review*, 5 [online]. Available from: https://www.equalrightstrust.org/ertdocumentbank/bob%20hepple.pdf

Horton, R. (2020, revised 2021) *The Covid-19 Catastrophe: What's Gone Wrong and How to Stop It Happening Again*, Cambridge: Polity Press.

Liberty (2019) *Hostile Environment*, London: Liberty [online]. Available from: https://www.libertyhumanrights.org.uk/fundamental/hostile-environment/#:~:text=Government%20has%20embedded%20immigration%20control,racist%20policies%20must%20be%20scrapped

Liverpool City Region (2021) 'A fairer, stronger, cleaner city region: where no one if left behind', *Liverpool City Region* [online]. Available from: https://www.liverpoolcityregion-ca.gov.uk/corporate-plan/

Mamluck, L. and Jones, T. (2020) *Rapid Review Exploring Disproportionate Impact of COVID-19 on Black, Asian and Minority Ethnic Communities*, Bristol: Applied Research Collaboration West.

Marmot, M. et al (2010) 'Fair society, healthy lives: the Marmot Review', Institute of Health Equity [online]. Available from: https://www.instituteofhealthequity.org/resources-reports/fair-society-healthy-lives-the-marmot-review

—— (2020) 'Build back fairer: the COVID-19 Marmot Review', Institute of Health Equity. Available from: http://www.instituteofhealthequity.org/resources-reports/build-back-fairer-the-covid-19-marmot-review

—— (2021) 'How a difficult childhood makes it more likely you'll have mental and physical problems as an adult', *The Conversation*, 23 April.

May, Theresa (2010) Theresa May's equality strategy speech (as written, not as delivered), Coin Street Community Centre, 17 November [online]. Available from: https://www.gov.uk/government/speeches/theresa-mays-equality-strategy-speech

Meaden, B. (2020) 'Liz Truss, Michel Foucault, and Leo Tolstoy', *Ecclesia*, 18 [online]. Available from: http://old.ekklesia.co.uk/node/30245

Munford, L. and Mott, L. et al (2022) *Overcoming Health Inequalities in Left Behind Neighbourhoods*, London: Local Trust for the All-Party Parliamentary Group (APPG) on Left Behind Neighbourhoods.

Murray, D. (2006) *Neoconservatism: Why We Need It*, London: Encounter Books.

Palmer, F. (1986) *Anti-Racism: An Assault on Education and Value*, London: Sherwood.

Pickett, K, et al (2021) *The Child of the North: Building a Fairer Future After COVID-19*, Lancaster: Northern Health Science Alliance (NHSA) and N8 Research Partnership.

Public Health England (2020) *Disparities in the Risks and Outcomes of COVID-19*, London: Public Health England.

Race Disparity Unit (2021) *Final Report on Progress to Address COVID-19 Health Inequalities*. London: HM Government. Available from: https://www.gov.uk/government/publications/final-report-on-progress-to-address-covid-19-health-inequalities

Razai, M. et al (2021a) 'Mitigating ethnic disparities in COVID-19 and beyond', *British Medical Journal*, 14 January [online]. Available from: doi: 10.1136/bmj.m4921.

—— (2021b) 'Structural racism is a fundamental cause and driver of ethnic disparities in health', *British Medical Journal*, 31 March [online]. Available from: https://blogs.bmj.com/bmj/2021/03/31/structural-racism-is-a-fundamental-cause-and-driver-of-ethnic-disparities-in-health/

Richardson, R. (2022) 'Education and equalities in Britain, 2010–2022: due regard and disregard in a time of pandemic', *London Review of Education*, 20(1): 22. doi: 10.14324/LRE.20.1.22

Roy, A. (2020) 'The pandemic is a portal', *Financial Times*, 3 April.

Royall, J. (2010) 'Socio-economic equality duty statement', House of Lords, 18 November [online]. Available from: https://www.theyworkforyou.com/lords/?id=2010-11-18a.914.1

Scottish Government (2018) *Fairer Scotland Duty: Interim Guidance for Public Bodies*, Edinburgh: Scottish Government.

Scruton, R. (2014) *How to be a Conservative*, London: Bloomsbury Continuum.

Singer, M. (2009) *Introduction to Syndemics: a Critical Systems Approach to Public and Community Health*, San Francisco, CA: Jossey-Bass.

Slack, J. (2010) 'Home Secretary Theresa May to axe Harmon's "ridiculous" equality law', *Daily Mail*, 17 November [online]. Available from: https://www.dailymail.co.uk/news/article-1330307/Theresa-May-axe-Harriet-Harmons-ridiculous-equality-law.html#comments

Tolhurst, A. (2020) 'Parts of a "bonkers" Liz Truss speech on equality were erased from the government website', Politics Home, 18 December [online]. Available from: https://www.politicshome.com/news/article/sections-of-a-liz-truss-speech-on-equality-erased-from-government-website-after-being-labelled-bonkers-and-gratuitous-provocation

Toynbee, P. (2009) 'Harman's law is Labour's biggest idea for 11 years', *The Guardian*, 13 January [online]. Available from: https://www.theguardian.com/commentisfree/2009/jan/13/polly-toynbee-harriet-harman-social-mobility.

Truss, E. (2020) 'The new fight for fairness', speech at the Centre for Policy Studies, London.

Villines, Z. (2020) 'What we know about racial traumas', Medical News Today, 22 July.

Webber, F. (2022) *Equalities, Free Expression and 'War on Woke'*, London: Institute of Race Relations.

Welsh Government (updated 2021) 'The socio-economic duty: guidance and resources for public bodies', Gov.Wales [online]. Available from: https://gov.wales/socio-economic-duty

Williams, J. (2021) *Rethinking Race: a Critique of Contemporary Anti-racism Programmes*, London: Civitas.

Wu, J. (2020) 'Racism's effects on Black mental health', *Psychology Today*, 7 October.

Younge, G. (2021) 'What COVID taught us about racism – and what we need to do now', *The Guardian*, 16 December.

NINE

Out of breath: intersections of inequality in a time of global pandemic

Anon

Introduction

Breathing is a function so fundamental to life that most of the time its significance goes unrecognised; yet the absence of the ability to breathe freely is a reality for many. The recent global COVID-19 pandemic – which particularly affects the lungs – has exposed an intersection of pandemic and capitalism in which some bodies are affected more than others; research findings show that people of the global majority have been disproportionately impacted by coronavirus (University of Manchester, 2020). Simultaneously, the death of George Floyd, and the pain of his final words, 'I can't breathe', has shown how the life-breath of some humans is more valued than that of others.

This chapter draws on bell hooks' (1994: 130) notion of critical dialogue; a practice that involves 'individuals who occupy different locations … mapping out terrains of commonality, connection and shared concern'. For hooks, coming together in the spirit of beloved community requires us to cross borders, thereby enriching each other's knowledge. As educators at either ends of the spectrum of privilege and oppression (Author A is a white female academic, and Author B an activist-writer of colour), we have used this dialogic space to explore the intersection of pandemic and inequality. By making the choice to write anonymously, we have also made a deliberate effort to detach from the ego associated with academic writing, and we invite others to adopt a similar dialogic model by which to converse as equals (privilege and structural inequalities notwithstanding).

We begin from a series of questions: Who is able to breathe? Why are some individuals afforded 'breathing space' and not others? What can we learn from the necropolitics of the pandemic (Mbembe and Corocoran, 2019), and how might we utilise this knowledge to take action for affirmative social change in education? We then explore the role of education in making change and conclude by reflecting on the role of dialogic processes in furthering and enriching understanding.

The right to breathe

A: The collision of the pandemic and the Black Lives Matter protests connects the idea of breath, and who is able to breathe. Shall we start by thinking about this collision and what it means?

B: You know that I often use an analogy about racism and oxygen – racism is part of the air that sustains us and, to shock you out of it, you need to hold your breath for a while. When you talk about breathing, for me it's more about having space. Having space to be free, to be. And racism takes that away from people, on both sides. People are so enamoured with the air we breathe; that is, the systems we are part of, that something like the virus was seen as being 'neutral'; everyone is equally affected. I said from the start that the manifestation of the virus is discriminatory, and people didn't want to hear this at first. Yet we know that groups are not only more vulnerable for systemic reasons but also due to issues of intergenerational trauma.

What we are seeing now with the COVID-19 vaccine is another complex issue that has been put forward as a neutral health intervention. And yet, generationally, there is huge trauma connected to the history of experiments on Black and Brown bodies. The Tuskegee Study, the disproportionate availability of the polio vaccine, the child-grabs from Indigenous and First Nations peoples, forced sterilisations by the state and so on. These violent medical events are in living memory, they are still happening now in many cases. It is no wonder that people of colour are anxious about this recent intervention that is being accepted without question.

The global North are, of course, profiteering as well; the vaccine is being held back and its use restricted via the refusal of waivers for the patent. Immunisation is talked about in neutral terms, yet medicine is imbued with power and profit, and is highly political.

A: This idea of neutrality crops up in academic research too; but research is a dirty word to many communities, particularly Indigenous nations who had research 'done to' them. It literally cannot be talked about because it caused such serious offence and harm. As Linda Tuhiwai Smith says: 'Research is inextricably linked to European imperialism and colonialism' (1999: 1). It has a really problematic and damaging history. And these conversations often fall into good/bad binaries as we don't take the time to carefully think through the complexities of ethics together.

B: This sums up how reductive the whole [COVID] debate is. Much like the debate around racism, we're continually led back to ideas of meritocracy; 'We're all in it together; we're all in the same boat.' And yet we're clearly not.

A: Can you say a little more about space in terms of racism and the pandemic? It has been a central concern from the start yet we rarely discuss who is afforded 'breathing space', the impact issues of overcrowding or lack of access to space, and what this means.

B: For me it's about **who** is able to breathe freely and be themselves in space. Everything is framed around the dominant culture being the norm. For example, would I be happy wearing a ceremonial *chanlo*, *Kurta* pyjama and *dhoti* walking into an organisational space? Absolutely not. And would my organisation be happy for me to speak Gujarati, Hindi, or Kiswahili? Because when English is your second or third language, it's tiring. You can't bring your whole self to the space, you have to leave stuff outside the door; because it's about survival. It's you tending towards whiteness, and that whiteness is: accent dropping; using a different dialect; making different lexical choices. It's wearing a suit. It's inhabiting spaces that you wouldn't normally inhabit, and that you wouldn't want to inhabit. It's believing and buying into policies and ideologies that don't necessarily serve you. This can be internalised as hate, or held up by a narrative of 'if I can do it, why can't you?' This takes no account of context and it's too reductive.

It pulls us to the idea that whiteness is the norm, whiteness is healthiness; and what this is doing in the current pandemic is killing people of colour and revealing stark inequities across the board.

A: I'm now thinking about space in relation to education and how everything is framed around the term 'inclusion'. This has become a meaningless watchword for equality, and yet it is essentially about inviting people to take a seat at a table which has already been set. Like you said, you might not still be able to be yourself or breathe freely. Because even though there purports to be a system of inclusion going on, there's still a box that people of colour have to fit into, because the system has not been designed for them. It's based around a certain idea of what it means to be human and, even though you might layer on these other aspects at the end of the day, the system design is fundamentally wrong. In fact, I switch off when I hear the word 'inclusion' now, because it is not about difference, it is about some normative framing and it is based around deficit.

B: I recently attended a poetry reading with Hodan Yusuf and Suhaiymah Manzoor-Khan (The Brown Hijabi). And in both their poems they talked about how you might have a seat at the table, but can you *speak* at the table? Can you *eat* at the table? So when we talk about inclusion, do we really mean inclusion; a situation where your voice is valued? When I take a seat at the table, am I able to represent my full self or am I forced to show a whitewashed version of myself? We need to think with Angela Davis; do we want real inclusion that means being part of a racist hetero-patriarchy? Why *would* we want that?

Thinking more widely, even with a shift to more egalitarian politics, we would still be in the same situation of capitalism that is rooted in an ideology that leads to the commodification of Black and Brown bodies (Mills, 1997). It is like the vaccine that has 95 per cent efficacy. The disease is still present. It can help to view racism through a pathogen-like lens; hostile bacteria, viruses and fungi are rarely beaten in their entirety. There are incidents of pathogens frozen in permafrost in a different form for millenia – only to arise when the environment is conducive to their growth. Racism may not be as overt, or in the form of physical violence, but the mutated strains, that is, racism in its different forms, are still as damaging.

And I do wonder how bad things need to get before we see proper change. How many people have to die before we stand up and say this is wrong? After George Floyd and numerous other Black lives have been taken by the authorities, we still persist in talking about the value of some lives and not others.

Education and activism

A: I think there is often talk about revolution, but you know me – I'm not a Marxist, and I often worry that we may continue to talk about a revolution that will never come. Rosi Braidotti always says that capitalism doesn't break; it bends (Bradiotti and Regan, 2017: 185). We see this fluidity in capitalism's constant shape-shifting, as it takes new territories; just look at the profiteering from the pandemic! The money being made from home-schooling, free school meals, protective equipment and vaccines … capitalism sees a space and quickly moves in. And we're completely embedded in it, in different ways and to different extents. Just this week I've been helping refugees from the Democratic Republic of the Congo, using the *self-same iPhone* which has had its parts mined for cobalt by child workers in that very country. It is difficult to reconcile my work as a volunteer with the way I am enmeshed in extractive capitalist regimes. But, of course, we don't operate outside of these systems; we're a part of them, and I think some people find this very hard to accept.

This linear idea of revolution; of reaching an endgame, an outcome, just leaves us in perpetual stasis and so perhaps it is more helpful to think about what we can do in the here and now. You often talk about revolution of the mind, so perhaps there is something here about education? Changing the paradigm and rethinking what it actually is for. Education is currently steeped in humanistic ideals that have excluded and 'othered' certain people over centuries, and is rooted in a normative framing of what 'human' is. If we can shift this – a kind of decolonisation of the mind – then starting with education may be the best way forward. Or am I being too simplistic?

B: With racism too, it's worth remembering that we benefit from the systems we are part of. Acknowledging the fact that we may benefit from racism, and that we're not just complicit; we're duplicitous, is all part of this educational awareness raising; 'conscientisation', as Paulo Freire (1985) would put it.

Decolonisation exists in the mind primarily. Each teacher does not live in a vacuum but comes to the table with an existing colonised view of the world. The first step is to challenge and interrogate one's ontological stance, as this is the basis of all learning; but, more importantly, the role of an educator is coterminously that of an epistemologist, artist and politician (Freire, 1985). As such, we cannot separate out these roles (and nor should we try to), but we need to consciously reflect on how we enact them every day.

It's exactly the same with racism and COVID; you can't look at these things in isolation, they are part of a whole. We need to broaden our lens, while at the same time drilling down into the minutiae. We need critical training; a new form of pedagogy – which moves away from reductionist thinking and mindless slogans towards more complexity and philosophical debate. This is the danger in the current education system where knowledge is commodified and yet no-one is able to critically appraise these atomised items and components of information.

A: We also need to spend more time examining our own positionality. There's very little professional development space for teachers – once qualified – to explore their values, histories and cultural understandings of education. Over here we often stigmatise therapy and counselling while it is culturally acceptable in countries like the US – and actually, why don't we engage more with these interventions on a professional level? Therapeutic practice would help us to explore, not only our personal histories but our relations to the world, to power, to the racialised spaces we find ourselves in.

B: Yes! Because with whiteness, we're taught that we live in a relative paradise, and we don't interrogate this nearly enough. Alana Lentin (2020) calls us to become 'racially literate' so that we are able to see what racism does and are able to talk about the issues with knowledge and depth of understanding. Without this practice of critical exploration, people think; it's not our fault, we didn't do anything. Instead, we should own our position, and really think about what that space means.

A: And I think this is helpful to do on an individual basis. When this exploration is done, it is usually done in groups – say on the topic of white privilege – where there isn't the space and time to properly explore pain. And by pain, I mean everybody's pain. Everyone will have some kind of history regarding this, and we could begin with Foucault's (1983: p.xiii) call to 'examine the fascist inside us all'; that is, our own love of power. Everyone has this to some degree, I know I do! To ask; what is our own experience of oppressing others, for example. This is very uncomfortable but it's a vital question.

And I think this discomfort is necessary, because the pain is there; regardless of whether we explore it or not. At least if we can look it in the face, we can then say – what can I do with this knowledge I now have? How can I take action?

B: It was Fanon in *The Wretched of the Earth* (2001) who said; decolonisation is always a violent act. This doesn't mean that the process is about physical violence. The epistemological viewpoint of educators will absolutely impact their pedagogy, so that they are caught in a miasma of power, sustaining itself through all those different bodies. That's why going to these places of discomfort is so important, so that teachers might gain awareness of their own limitations and seek out ways to read the world differently.

A: It really helps to look at issues through different ethical lenses too. During COVID we have only seen things from a utilitarian viewpoint, rooted in a worship of the economy; and we're back to colonialism and commodification once again. What happens if we were to take a different ethical frame – say a feminist ethic of care, for example? That might lead us to look differently at decision-making, and say that perhaps, for this individual who is dying, it is best that they see their family this Christmas.

B: Absolutely; the framing of ethical practice and thought is the crux of all societal oppression. It's interesting that you mention a feminist ethic of care. John Stuart Mill in his (1869) essay *The Subjection of Women* wrote about and supported rights for women. From the perspective of an anti-oppressive activist, this gets a thumbs up from me. However, no thought or ideology exists in a vacuum. Mill and Bentham famously advocated utilitarianism and followed the Malthusian principle. We need this context to see how their concepts were based around a classed and racialised understanding of the world and have led to blame being put on the poorest people for the world's problems.

A: Yes, we don't question the ethical systems that we live by nearly enough; and are rarely taught ethics. So we don't know that, say, many Indigenous communities use entirely different ethical systems. Or that there are other moral frameworks, based around relationships rather than individuals and their dispositions. We find it impossible to even begin to comprehend that other ways of doing things might actually be possible.

B: This is the space that education needs to fill, I think! Making the classroom a 'space of radical possibility' (hooks, 1994: 12) so that we can always strive to be better.

Dialogue

A: There is so much to discuss, and we've only begun to scratch the surface. I feel like we've really explored the complexity of our current predicament and started to make important connections between the key issues of pandemic and racism. There's lots of work to do.

Conversations like the one we have had today can be really generative and a good starting point; they allow us to get to the heart of ethical concerns without becoming rooted in binary viewpoints. David Bohm (1996: 6) talks about dialogue being a 'stream of meaning, flowing among and through us and between us'. I would like to thank you for creating new meaning with me today, and for teaching me a huge amount.

B: Thank you. You are amazing. Nearly all learning is a social act! (Black and Allen, 2007). And I am richer for our conversation.

References

Black, S. and Allen, J. (2007) 'Part 5: learning is a social act', *The Reference Librarian*, 59(2): 76–91.

Bohm, D. (1996) *On Dialogue,* London: Routledge.

Braidotti, R. and Regan, L. (2017) 'Our times are always out of joint: feminist relational ethics in and of the world today: an interview with Rosi Braidotti', *Women: A Cultural Review*, 28(3): 171–192.

Foucault, M. (1983) 'Preface', in G. Deleuze and F. Guattari (eds), R. Hurley, M. Seem and H.R. Lane (trans), *Anti-Oedipus*, London: Bloomsbury Academic, pp xi–xiv.

Freire, P. (1985) 'Reading the world and reading the word: an interview with Paulo Freire', *Language Arts*, 62(1): 15–21.

hooks, b. (1994) *Teaching to Transgress: Education as the Practice of Freedom*, New York: Routledge.

Lentin, A. (2020) *Why Race Still Matters*, London: Polity Press.

Mbembe, A. and Corcoran, S. (2019) *Necropolitics*, London: Duke University Press.

Mill, J.S. (1869) *The Subjection of Women,* London: Longmans, Green, Reader and Dyer.

Mills, C. (1997) *The Racial Contract*, New York: Cornell University Press.

Tuhiwai Smith, L. (1999) *Decolonising Methodologies: Research and Indigenous Peoples*, London: University of Otago Press.

TEN

An exploration of the label 'BAME' and other existing collective terminologies, and their effect on mental health and identity within a COVID-19 context

Ibiyemi Moshie-Moses

Introduction

The limited literature on the topic of collective terminology has had a resurgence since the COVID-19 outbreak, highlighting the issues with current terms and the need for change (Aspinall 2002; 2020). The year 2020 tested people on every continent – and not only because of COVID-19. The outbreak of the virus tested our physical health, our health systems, our governments, our economies, our collective mental health, our patience and our limits as human beings. The introduction of new language has tested our adaptability. The terms decolonise, white privilege and racial disparities are almost as popular as tiers, social distancing and PPE, when discussing the virus, making the link between COVID-19 and racism undoubtable. The effects of COVID-19 have unified us as humans sharing the same uncertain experience; however, it has not affected us equally.

COVID-19 has highlighted inequalities showing that UK 'BAME' (Black, Asian and Minority Ethnic) communities are dying at higher rates (Bhala et al, 2020) than communities racialised as white British. While devastating, the pandemic has magnified the fragmentation of our society, bringing buried prejudices and years of systemic racism into sharper view. The use of collective terms during this pandemic and the subsequent broadcasting of statistics to the general public has, unsurprisingly, brought issues with labelling closer to the fore. In a discussion about racial language between Lincoln's Bar and Judiciary members, Thomas QC says, 'whatever you label us is not the issue, the issue is how we are treated' (Shotunde Sidhu and Thomas, 2020). Payne (2013: 394) sees 'all aspects of identity as profoundly and intrinsically socially produced', so if our labels infer otherness or imply derogation this will likely have a direct effect on the collective identity of people with a non-European heritage, and in turn the individual's mental health within these groups. Therefore, although 'how we are treated' is paramount, its salience need not be distinguished from 'whatever you label us', for they are one and the same, and both have the power to affect identity.

While analysing the literature available on the subject of racialised descriptors, the need for systematic consideration of these terms became evident. As the government research and assign such terms that define millions, and the statistics show that BAME communities are underrepresented in the UK government (Uberoi and Lees, 2020), it becomes plain that a framework is needed to assist governmental bodies with this weighted task. This will ensure that in these highly stressful times, labels that have the power to affect identity so directly are being thoroughly considered. This research has developed a framework revealing the main requirements that ethnic labels should embody, while keeping in mind a consciousness framed in decoloniality. The latter part of this chapter will discuss CALC (Compassion, Accuracy, Linguistic, Context), which calculates the least flawed term according to the research available.

The popular argument regarding the label 'BAME' in relation to COVID-19 is the 'lack of specificity' in the acronym when analysing COVID-19 data (Milner and Jumbe, 2020: e419). 'BAME' covers innumerable ethnicities with different lifestyles. To disregard the variety within 'BAME' reduces millions of people's experiences to a single one, and in terms of COVID-19 research and data the results are bound to be vague and inaccurate when generalising in this way. Sze et al (2020) also take issue with the ambiguity of the language and suggest a more standardised approach across disciplines in order to shine a light on specific systemic problems. Milner and Jumbe (2020) argued that an intersectional approach must be adopted to fully understand COVID-19 disparities between ethnic groups. By removing the 'catch all' (Aspinall, 2002: 804) term and instead using specific descriptors the groups most affected could be identified by. Aldridge et al (2020: 3) took this approach in their research and found:

> The largest total number of deaths in minority ethnic groups were Indian (492 deaths) and Black Caribbean (460 deaths) people ... There was no statistical evidence that SMRs (standardised mortality ratios) were increased or reduced for Chinese, Mixed White and Black African, Mixed White and Asian, and Mixed White and Black Caribbean ethnic groups.

This reveals that the use of the vague term BAME when discussing COVID-19 statistics is unhelpful, as ethnicities within this umbrella term are differently affected. Though BAME is convenient it 'unhelpfully blends ethnicity, geography, nationality – and in doing so erases our identity and reduces us to an Other' (#BAMEOver, 2020: n.p.). Another form of othering is the 'unnecessary emphasis on skin colour'

(Afridi and Warmington, 2009: 6). The descriptor 'Black', once widely accepted, is now dividing the community. Some feel proud to use the reclaimed word to describe themselves, whereas others deem it a derogatory term centering the imagined social construct of race and promoting prejudice and racism (Tsri, 2015).

Campaigns such as TAOBQ (The African Or Black Question) argue that replacing Black with African is the necessary move to progress in anti-'Afriphobic' activism and support the use of AAME (African, Asian and Minority Ethnic) (Kwaku, 2011). Such campaigns and the continued contestation from within the Black community exemplifies the variety of identifications within this homogenously presented group.

Despite its problems, Aspinall (2020) reveals that BME (Black and Minority Ethnic) has been used on official records and in parliament since 1987. In academic and political circles, it is well established and has become semantically versatile; public health agencies use BME as adjectives and nouns (Aspinall, 2020). This convenience is supported by BAME's introduction into the *Oxford English Dictionary* in 2014. Despite wide usage of BME and BAME in certain circles, in 2019: 'Research undertaken by the government's Race Disparity Audit, on the use of terminology relating to ethnicity, found that among nearly 300 people across the UK, only two (<1%) recognized the acronyms, and only one knew in general terms what they stood for' (Aspinall, 2020: 6). Knowing this, it is not surprising that 'few of the people referred to with this label see it as an appropriate description of their identity' (Richardson, 2006: 6). Thus, we recognise the absence of interest convergence which posits that 'the interest of blacks in achieving racial equality will be accommodated only when it converges with the interests of whites' (Bell, 1980: 523). Continued use of a term that fails to reach the very people it refers to, and instead circulates within the power structures, threatens to ostracise communities even further from a government that already does not represent them (Uberoi and Lees, 2020).

Richardson (2006) is shocked at the mechanistic, narrow use of an acronym to describe groups of people. Since the colonisation of Africa, this dehumanising language resulting in degradation, has been the main tool of subjugation and the justification of the racist and capitalist hierarchies that remain in place in the global North. One way this pervasive and long-standing British belief has been reaffirmed is in the over policing of the racialised other (Long, 2018). Since Black people are 43 times more likely to be stopped by police outside of London, it is fair to assume that there may be anxieties surrounding belief in our governmental bodies (Liberty, 2020). This is officially untaught and avoided, yet quietly and continuously inferred, legacy of dehumanisation in Britain causes ostracisation, mistrust and fear – culminating in mental oppression.

Although the Cabinet Office advertise an anti-'BAME' position, this advice is not complied with throughout government (Aspinall, 2020). So why are the government misleading the public in their actions and attitudes on the topic of BAME? Lawler (2008: 10) believes that 'Westerners' tend 'to see identities as finished products rather than as active, processual engagements within the social world'. The results of this attitude are explored in more recent work by Yep and Lescure (2019: 120) in *Thick Intersectionality,* where it is found that 'thinking of identity as a being tends to foreclose engaging with its complexity and fluidity. Thinking of identity as a becoming, however, allows for it to be understood more fluidly and expansively'. This 'fixed' identity that Frantz Fanon (1952) explored 50 years previous in his seminal work *Black Skin, White Masks* restricts entire communities from progression and development. This long-standing paradigm continues to permeate societal readings of identity, stunting growth and disabling progress. Unwillingness from the government to candidly debunk BAME is evidence of the battle in identity politics and of interest convergence.

Issue has been taken against BAME and BME for the past two decades (Aspinall, 2002). However, with the pandemic comes a greater demand to take responsibility and action, as this homogenisation and vagueness has the power to influence perceptions of mortality rates.

One phrase has made its way across the Atlantic where it is used as a collective term for mainly African American and Latinx communities. People Of Colour (POC) made its debut in American legislation in 1803 where it was 'employed as an … exclusionary device for oppression of those deemed "of color"' (Elengold, 2015: 26). By adopting the American phrase, we unconsciously compare and strengthen our connection to their struggle. And, while there are obvious similarities concerning racial injustices, the modern, cultural and historical contexts are very different (McIntosh and Owolade, 2020). Population estimates in July 2019 showed that while the white population still occupied the vast majority, as in the UK, the population of POC was much higher in the US, seeing 18.5 per cent for Hispanic or Latinx, 13.4 per cent African American and 5.9 per cent for Asian communities (US Census Bureau, 2019). Asian groups were bigger in the UK at 6.8 per cent; however, Black communities made up less than 10 per cent of the population (IRR, 2011). Owolade (2020) exemplifies the difference between Black communities in the UK to the US by highlighting that most of the population in the UK are descended from migrants, whereas the majority of the population in the US are 'descended from the victims of the transatlantic slave trade … so we have two significantly different Black populations'. Because of this, both communities have nuanced and specific struggles. To use a one-size-fits-all method for collective terminologies across the global North, ignores the diversity between cultures and implies that our nuances are standardised across the globe. This subtracts from the individual's experience by reducing international communities to essentialist stereotypes, homogenising millions of people. These generalisations are bound to have a confusing effect on identity and raise concerns in a modern-day context where the current crisis benefits from ambiguity.

Another issue with the term People Of Colour is that it ignores the disadvantages and prejudices faced by white ethnic communities such as Romani people, Gypsies and Travellers as highlighted by Aspinall (2020) when discussing the term BAME. The effects on these communities from COVID-19 have gone largely unexamined (Heaslip and Parker, 2020). While concerns have been raised to the likely disproportionate impact COVID-19 will have on Gypsy and Roma Traveller communities due to existing 'health inequalities', figures remain hidden beneath vague terminology from the NHS and Public Health England's data. According to Citizens Advice (2010: n.p.) race discrimination occurs 'if you're treated unfairly because of … color, nationality, ethnic origin or national origin'. In terms of attainment, these white ethnic groups have been found to have more disadvantaged experiences of the schooling system compared to any other group of children, with Roma children's achievement reaching 50 per cent or less than that of their Indian, Chinese, Black, mixed, and white British counterparts (Department for Education, 2020). A term that considers these groups when discussing disparities and disadvantages seems necessary.

The phrase is useful linguistically, considering intersectionality (Crenshaw, 1989). The noun can be swapped and, for example, Women of Colour or Queer People of Colour's individual problems and disadvantages can be targeted. The term has been critiqued after a survey was taken, however, revealing that 'in the UK for many people over 35 this has uncomfortable resonance with the racist terminology "coloureds"' (#BAMEOver, 2020). The lack of empathy encapsulated in the term is not the most suitable descriptor to use during this global crisis when 'among the general population, COVID-19 transmission fear has facilitated the development of psychiatric symptoms such as depression, confusion, stress and anxiety among individuals who have never previously experienced mental illness' (Khan et al, 2020: 2). They go on to say that people 'may also blame one another and develop aggressive behavior towards people who are ill or perceived as ill' (2). With media asserting that People Of Colour are affected disproportionately by COVID-19, the added pressure of accusation on top of oppressive language being normalised in a time when language and specificity directly impacts morbidity, could cause further dissociation from society impacting POC's mental health dangerously.

Minority Ethnic is often used as the most neutral collective term (Aspinall, 2020; Bhala et al, 2020; Uberoi and Lees, 2020). While Minority Ethnic or Ethnic Minority (as the terms are often used interchangeably) takes a 'colour-free' stance, linguistically there is much about the term that implies Otherness (Afridi and Warmington, 2009: 6). 'Minority' Richardson (2006: 6) reveals 'in many places in Britain … is mathematically inaccurate or misleading'; certainly globally it is inaccurate. This distribution of unreliable data about ethnic minority populations has long been a marker of British society whether overt or subliminal. The assignment of Blackness onto the 'Black' body instead of brownness, which is more accurate, connotes from the outset that the Black body is related to sin and everything unholy and tarred 'sin is black as virtue is white' (Fanon, 1952: 118). This systematic othering has become the global norm. The modern antidote to this Afro pessimism or 'Afriphobia' (Kwaku, 2011) are movements like Black is Beautiful, which has been altering the connotations of Blackness since the 1960s, and the Black Lives Matter (BLM) movement, which remind society that Black skin is not a weapon. 'Inaccurate or misleading' information sewn into common parlance further reifies integrally racist ideas and allows them to permeate society at all levels affecting ethnic minority communities' image and identity. Fanon (1952) asks how can the Black man think anything but negatively of himself when Black is represented as sin? These movements are, therefore, necessary to decolonise the language surrounding, and liberate the minds of, ethnic minority populations as well as our counterparts racialised as white.

The use of the term 'minority' as a human descriptor is a dampener for Minority Ethnic communities, suggesting smallness, limited capacity, a subtle controlling restraint on the minds of the people it describes. Fanon's (1952: 165) interpretation of Jung's theory of the 'collective unconscious' is that it is not 'inherited cerebral matter' regarding genetics, 'the collective unconscious is quite simply the repository of prejudices, myths and collective attitudes of a particular group'. This denial of the biological in favour of the sociological brings attention to individual psychological states. These lexiconic implications evidence the second principle of white supremacy (Ansley, 1997). Growing up in a society where whiteness is hegemonic, constantly hearing 'prejudices' 'of a particular group' can result in a complicated relationship with the self for Minority Ethnic people adding to the complex, prejudice collective unconscious of society today.

The term 'ethnic' is used to refer only to those who are thought to differ from some assumed indigenous norm of 'Britishness' (Payne, 2013: 110). Payne goes on to mention the '"ethnic look" in the world of fashion', and 'ethnic cuisine', while Richardson (2006: 6) talks of 'ethnic teachers' and 'ethnic children'. Using the word as a noun has been interpreted as 'seriously depersonalising and offensive' and it is more readily accepted when used in conjunction with minority and validated with humanising terms such as 'communities' or 'people' (Richardson, 2006: 6). These phrases homogenise and 'Orientalise' anything typically 'non-British' and, with it, exoticise the imagined places they come from (Said, 1978). This exotification dehumanises people, reducing a human being to an 'ethnic' token, a means of entertainment and curiosity to the hegemonic populous. Thus, the term Ethnic Minority could be critiqued as both limiting and othering.

Canada's preferred collective phrase, 'Visible Minorities', has appeared in the UK. This colour-blind approach seeks to end racism by simply not speaking about it. Lorde (1984) discusses this strategy of ignorance claiming that individuals are taught to fear what we do not understand. This manifests in three ways: ignoring the issue, translating to colour-blindness; copying it, which results in the commodification of Blackness; or destroying it, which takes form in the binary narrative that is created – white is good, Black is bad, to vastly oversimplify. This denial of racism, or 'colour-blind racism' that modern society adopts, causes further traumas to visible minorities and can result in 'gaslighting', causing victims to feel mentally unstable and question their capacity (Tobias and Joseph, 2018). Agreeing that we live in a 'post-race' society denies the experiences of 14 per cent of the UK population (Bhala et al, 2020) resulting in the gaslighting of entire communities in the UK. This is supported by the mental health sectioning statistics by ethnicity, in England from 2018–2019 (National Statistics, 2019). This psychological manipulation within society added to the strain of systemic racism calls for the decolonisation of language. At best, this phrase is naive; at worst, it is consciously muting conversations on race to maintain white supremacy and discourage any open, honest discourse surrounding the topic, furthering the argument against imported terminologies. While using visible ethnic minority as his preferred term, Sidhu QC remarks in concern to outward racism, that 'although those who are perpetrating that sort of menace within our society don't spend too much time making a distinction between whether you are Brown or Black, if you are of a different colour to them, and they are white, that is the principle distinction that they draw' (Shotunde, Sidhu and Thomas, 2020). This learned prejudice historically also had a detrimental effect on the white population's mental health, as explored by Cesaire (2000). Sidhu could be at risk of recentering whiteness and prioritising white comfort when determining terminology that concerns all but the population who are racialised as white. By centralising narratives of overt acts of racism, this also fails to bring the insidiousness of systemic racism to the fore and gives the term racism a one-dimensionality that is best avoided. In order to decolonise language, the centering of the voices of visible minority communities must be acted upon; this example fails in that respect (Rollock and Gillborn, 2011). Some prefer this term because of the avoidance of 'colour' or 'race,' however, as well as existing contention with the word minorities, it could be argued that the use of the word 'visible' still promotes Othering through aesthetic appearance. This term includes white visible minority groups, who, as a critique to many of the existing terminologies, are often left out (Afridi and Warmington, 2009), even though they suffer from similar disadvantages in concern to schooling and prejudice as previously discussed.

Some researchers advising abandonment of current terms are offering original alternatives. In this next section these alternate collective terminologies will be discussed and dissected using the critical CALC framework to predict their potential success today. This analysis is not exhaustive and acts as a trial exercise to explore whether a framework would be beneficial to such a governmental decision-making process as choosing collective terminologies.

Many of the issues with the current terminologies were based on a lack of *COMPASSION* for the people that they define, often forgetting that beyond the statistics were human beings with complicated identities, feelings and histories. *ACCURACY* ensures that the groups being presented are the specific groups that the information is about, and the information therefore valid. By ensuring accuracy, blending 'ethnicity, geography, nationality' will be avoided intentionally (#BAMEOver, 2020: n.p.). The next section considers whether the term is grammatically correct, is versatile in its *LINGUISTIC* usage, and is adaptable on different platforms, for example in activist movements, social media and the news. Finally, C stands for *CONTEXT*. For example, the term 'coloured', which was used widely historically, is deemed offensive today (Smith, 1992). Context also considers the modern mediums and popular topics that inform race discourse today. Recognition stemming from Twitter hash tags, social justice movements and activism could ensure the terms wide usage and comprehension.

Racialised minorities

Black British Academics deem 'minorities' 'a term that places non-white people in a subordinate position to those racialised as white'; the group, nevertheless, promotes 'Racialised Minorities' (Gabriel, 2013). Overall, though 'Racialised Minorities' succeeds as a political statement, and is revolutionary in highlighting the action committed, drawing attention to the racialisation of people of colour, it is more lacking, based on the CALC framework, than it is successful. This is due to the lack of compassion in the implication of the term 'minority', mentally marginalising and upholding social hierarchies, thus continuing colonial damage. The phrase continues the topical centralisation of 'race' discourse; however, academising 'race' talk could alienate people, stifling 'race' rhetoric and progress. This impenetrability of academia and its monopoly on knowledge has been critiqued as a remnant of Eurocentric colonial attitudes (Mirza, 2018; Pimblott, 2020).

Racially minoritised

A variation of the above is 'Racially Minoritised'. This term was introduced during the COVID-19 outbreak in response to statistics that show Racially Minoritised people dying at a considerably higher rate than white people (Bhala et al, 2020). Alongside the introduction of the term are suggestions on other language that ought to be used when discussing COVID-19. The use of the term 'white privilege' is promoted and authors 'suggest continued use of the word racism when discussing COVID-19 racial health disparities' (Milner and Jumbe, 2020: e.419). They also propose that 'the term ... confirms that so-called minoritisation is a social process, shaped by power', the conscious use of 'Minoritised' brings attention to this process, similar to 'Racialised' (Milner and Jumbe, 2020: e.419). However, though the word 'minoritised' was coined in 2003, it is not well known even within scholarly circles (Milner and Jumbe, 2020: e.419). This linguistic nuance could alienate those it seeks to liberate. Faring well in its compassion, the term struggles overall with its convenience, holding no space linguistically for specificity or intersectionality.

People who experience racism/PoWER

This term is one championed by the #BAMEOver (2020) movement, which utilised surveys as primary research to gauge what people who experience racism prefer to be described as and, more specifically, what they did not find appropriate. An adaptation of this, coined by Marcus Ryder, is the same term acronymised – 'PoWER'. Ryder (@marcusryder, 2020) proposes that PoWER could be specified by the relevant noun, for example 'you would have Black People Who Experience Racism – #BlackPoWER', '#WomanPoWER', '#GayPoWER'. PoWER speaks to younger generations, complimenting the narration of social justice and organisation of anti-racist movements through social media. There is a risk that the acronymisation of the phrase could result in meaning being lost reproducing BAME's incomprehension (Aspinall, 2020).

The likelihood of the government's official adoption of the term must also be considered and, given today's context with Race Disparity officials stating, 'much of the supposed evidence of institutional racism is flimsy' (Speare-Cole, 2020), realistically this phrase is too progressive to be adopted officially within the current zeitgeist.

Conclusion

PoWER performed best in the framework, however faltered in its Compassion – its acronymisation and the centralisation of demeaning experiences overshadowed its positive attributes for me personally, revealing the framework to be less methodical than anticipated. Though Racially Minoritised had many flaws through the CALC framework, it is identified as the most Compassionate. However, as PoWER centered the opinions of people with non-European heritage in its conception, and with the knowledge that one collective term will never be agreed upon by such a heterogeneous amalgamation of individuals, this could be more readily accepted as the preferred collective term revealing, perhaps, the most salient quality, which is the centering of the voices of the people the term describes. 'The fact is, all such labels are unsatisfactory and tend to be used as a matter of convenience until a better or less contested term takes their place' (Afridi and Warmington, 2009: 6). The current terms are highly contested and, considering the context of the moment, with the Black Lives Matter movement highlighting the disproportionate prejudice and stereotyping of Black people, and the subsequent frustration, fear and sadness that looms because of this, a change is overdue. In medical and clinical racial categorisations, it is imperative that specificity is attained, as the homogenisation of these groups continues to affect morbidity through COVID-19. This framework is one method that aims to label groups respectfully and accurately, while the labelling remains necessary. Further research into the areas of media journalism and social media are encouraged to provide a broader and deeper account of the collective terminologies used today and reactions to them. These are areas that require a separate focused analysis to improve cross-sectional accuracy, as this chapter has mainly looked at current academic literature. To keep the framework relevant, not only will new terms need to be added, but also the classifications updated as language and identities evolve in new contexts. What becomes evident is that the objective answer that the framework aims for is indeterminable due to the subjective nature of the topic and interpretivist direction of this chapter acknowledging that reality is determined by individual experience (Kivunja and Kuyini, 2017). This suggests accepting a majority consensus as sufficient, which 'BAME' (of which fewer than 1 per cent of people understand) has not (Aspinall, 2020). The nature of language is transient, as it evolves with the people that use it. Being able to best utilise language is about being open to and adaptable to the evolution of identity.

References

@marcusryder (2020) 'PoWER', *Twitter*, 27 June [online]. Available from https://twitter.com/marcusryder/status/1276697929495937024

#BAMEOver (2020) 'The #BAMEOver Live Debate', *Inc Arts UK* [online]. Available from: https://incarts.uk/%23bameover-the-statement

Afridi, A. and Warmington, J. (2009) *The Pied Piper: The BME Third Sector and the UK Race Relations Policy*, Birmingham: brap.

Aldridge, R.W., Lewer, D., Katikireddi, S.V., Mathur, R., Pathak, N., Burns, R., Fragaszy, E.B., Johnson, A.M., Devakumar, D., Abubakar, I. and Hayward, A. (2020) 'Black, Asian and Minority Ethnic groups in England are at increased risk of death from COVID-19: indirect standardisation of NHS mortality data', *Wellcome Open Research*, 5(88): 1–20. doi: 10.12688/wellcomeopenres.15922.2

Ansley, F.L. (1997). 'White supremacy (and what we should do about it)', in R. Delgado and J. Stefancic (eds), *Critical White Studies: Looking Behind the Mirror*, Philadelphia, PA: Temple University Press, pp 592–595.

Aspinall, P.J. (2002) 'Collective terminology to describe the minority ethnic population: the persistence of confusion and ambiguity in usage', *Sociology*, 36(4): 1–14.

Aspinall, P.J. (2020) 'ethnic/racial terminology as a form of representation: a critical review of the lexicon of collective and specific terms in use in Britain', *Genealogy,* 4(87): 1–14. doi: 10.3390/genealogy4030087

Bell, D.A. (1980) 'Brown v. Board of Education and the interest-convergence dilemma', *Harvard Law Review*, 93(3): 518–533.

Bhala, N., Curry, G., Martineau, A.R., Agyemang, C. and Bhopal, R. (2020) 'Sharpening the global focus on ethnicity and race in the time of COVID-19', *Lancet,* 395 (10238): 1673–1676.

Cesaire, A.F.D. (2000) *Discourse on Colonialism: A Poetics of Anticolonialism*, New York: Monthly Review Press.

Citizens Advice (2010) 'Gypsies and travellers – Race Discrimination', *National Association of Citizens Advice Bureaux* [online]. Available from: https://www.citizensadvice.org.uk/law-and-courts/discrimination/protected-characteristics/gypsies-and-travellers-race-discrimination/

Crenshaw, K. (1989) 'Demarginalizing the intersection of race and sex: a Black feminist critique of antidiscrimination doctrine, feminist theory and antiracist politics', *University of Chicago Legal Forum,* 1: 139–167.

Department for Education (2020) 'Percentage of 4 to 5 year olds who met the expected standard in development, by ethnicity', Gov.uk [online]. Available from: https://www.ethnicity-facts-figures.service.gov.uk/education-skills-and-training/early-years/attainment-of-development-goals-by-children-aged-4-to-5-years/latest

Elengold, K.S. (2015) 'Branding identity', *Denver Law Review,* 93(1): 1–53.

Fanon, F. (1952) *Black Skin, White Masks*, translated from French by C.L. Markmann, US: Grove Press.

Gabriel, D. (2013) 'Racial categorisation and terminology', *Black British Academics* [online]. Available from: https://blackbritishacademics.co.uk/about/racial-categorisation-and-terminology/

Heaslip, V. and Parker, J. (2020) The hidden impact of Coronavirus on gypsy, Roma travellers', *Conversation Trust* [online]. Available from: https://theconversation.com/the-hidden-impact-of-coronavirus-on-gypsy-roma-travellers-141015

Institute of Race Relations (IRR) (2011) 'Ethnicity and religion statistics', *Institute of Race Relations* [online]. Available from https://irr.org.uk/research/statistics/ethnicity-and-religion/

Khan, K.S., Mamun, M.A., Griffiths, M.D. and Ullah, I. (2020) 'The mental health impact of the COVID-19 pandemic across different cohorts', *International Journal of Mental Health and Addiction*, July: 1–7. doi: 10.1007/s11469-020-00367-0

Kivunja, C. and Kuyini, A.B. (2017) 'Understanding and Applying Research Paradigms in Educational Contexts', *International Journal of Higher Education*, 6(5): 26–41. doi: 10.5430/ijhe.v6n5p26

Kwaku (2011) 'About us: the African Or Black Question (TAOBQ) questioning what we call ourselves as people of African heritage in Britain', *Blogspot* [online]. Available from: taobq.blogspot.com/p/home.html

Lawler, S. (2008) *Identity: Sociological Perspectives*, UK: Polity Press.

Liberty (2020) 'Stop and search', *Liberty Human Rights* [online]. Available from: https://www.libertyhumanrights.org.uk/fundamental/stop-and-search/

Long, L.J. (2018) *Perpetual Subjects: A Critical Race Theory of Black and Mixed-Race Experiences of Policing*, UK: Palgrave MacMillan.

Lorde, A. (1984) *Sister Outsider*, New York: Crossing Press.

McIntosh, K. and Owolade, T. (2020) 'Across the red line: are American approaches to combating racism worth trying in Britain', *BBC*, November [online]. Available from: https://www.bbc.co.uk/sounds/play/m000p1g4

Milner, A. and Jumbe, S. (2020) 'Using the right words to address racial disparities in COVID-19', *Lancet*, 5: e419–e420. doi: 10.1016/S2468-2667(20)30162-6

Mirza, H.S. (2018) *Dismantling Higher Education: Racism, Whiteness and Decolonising the Academy*, US: Springer International Publishing.

National Statistics (2019) 'Mental Health Act statistics, annual figures 2018–19', *NHS Digital* [online]. Available from: https://digital.nhs.uk/data-and-information/publications/statistical/mental-health-act-statistics-annual-figures/2018-19-annual-figures

Owolade, T. (2020) 'Please stop imposing American views about race on us' [online]. Available from: https://www.persuasion.community/p/please-stop-imposing-american-views

Payne, G. (2013) *Social Divisions*, 3rd edn, UK: Palgrave Macmillan.

Pierce, M., Hope, H., Ford, T., Hatch, S., Hotopf, M., John, A., Kontopantelis, R.W., Wessely, S., McManus, S. and Abel, K.M. (2020) 'Mental health before and during the COVID-19 pandemic: a longitudinal probability sample survey of the UK population', *Lancet Psychiatry*, 7: 883–892. [online]. Available from: https://www.thelancet.com/journals/lanpsy/article/PIIS2215-0366(20)30308-4/fulltext

Pimblott, K. (2020) 'Decolonising the university: the origins and meaning of a movement', *The Political Quarterly,* 91(1): 210–216.

Richardson, R. (2006) 'To BME or not to BME? Questions, notes and thoughts about language, again', *Race Equality Teaching*, 25(1): 11–16.

Rollock, N. and Gillborn, D. (2011) *Critical Race Theory (CRT)*, UK: British Educational Research Association [online]. Available from https://www.bera.ac.uk/publication/critical-race-theory-crt

Said, E.W. (1978) *Orientalism*, US: Pantheon Books.

Shotunde, N., Sidhu, J. and Thomas, L. (2020) Lincoln's Inn panel discussion: 'Bar, BAME and COVID-19: a conversation that needs to be had', *YouTube*, June [online]. Available from: https://www.youtube.com/watch?v=ycBvTwj5K2o&feature=emb_title

Smith, T.W. (1992) 'Changing racial labels: from "Colored" to "Negro" to "Black" to "African American"', *Public Opinion Quarterly*, 56(4): 496–514.

Speare-Cole, R. (2020) 'Criticism over Tony Sewell heading government race commission after "flimsy" institutional racism comment', *Evening Standard*, 16 July [online]. Available from: https://www.standard.co.uk/news/politics/tony-sewell-government-race-commission-criticism-a4500521.html

Sze, S., Pan, D. Nevill, C.R., Gray, L.J., Martin, C.A., Nazareth, J., Minhas, J.S., Divall, P., Khunti, K., Abrams, K.R., Nellums, L.B. and Pareek, M. (2020) 'Ethnicity and clinical outcomes in COVID-19: a systematic review and meta-analysis', *Eclinical Medicine*, 29 (100630): 1–17. doi: 10.1016/j.eclinm.2020.100630

Tippett, N., Wolke, D. and Platt, L. (2013) 'Ethnicity and bullying involvement in a national UK youth sample', *Elsevier: Journal of Adolescence*, 36: 639–649. [online]. Available from: 10.1016/j.adolescence.2013.03.013

Tobias, H. and Joseph, A. (2018) 'Sustaining systemic racism through psychological gaslighting: denials of racial profiling and justifications of carding by police utilizing local news media', *Sage*, 10(4): 424–455. doi: 10.1177/2153368718760969

Tsri, K. (2015) 'Africans are not black: why the use of the term "black" for Africans should be abandoned', *African Identities*, 14(2): 147–160. doi: 10.1080/14725843.2015.1113120

Uberoi, E. and Lees, R. (2020) 'Ethnic diversity in politics and public life', *UK Parliament* [online]. Available from https://commonslibrary.parliament.uk/research-briefings/sn01156/

United States Census Bureau (2019) 'Quick facts United States', *United States Census Bureau* [online]. Available from https://www.census.gov/quickfacts/fact/table/US#

Yep, G.A. and Lescure, R. (2019) 'A thick intersectional approach to microaggressions', *Southern Communication Journal*, 84(2): 113–126. doi: 10.1080/1041794X.2018.1511749

ELEVEN

COVID-19 in the UK: a colour-blind response

Jane Hinchcliffe

As a young adult I was a subscriber to the idea of a colour-blind[1] society. I believed in the equality and diversity agenda of New Labour. I had a stock answer for equality questions in interviews (something about treating everyone fairly, but responding to individual needs) and I thought that colonialism and the Jim Crow era of US segregation were well and truly in the past. It takes a lot of unlearning of what you thought you knew to move forwards from there. I did not realise at the time that this was a colour-blind approach to racism, and that my belief in meritocracy was harmful.

Colour-blindness is the practice of not seeing, or claiming not to see, colour or race. It situates racism firmly on the margins, with overt racists. Public discourse is around equality for all, but colour is seen and used as a tool for discrimination in private (Gotanda, 1991). The colour-blind view ignores or conceals the impact of hundreds of years of white supremacist thinking on laws, policy and society (Annamma, Jackson and Morrison, 2016).

With the rise of Black Lives Matter worldwide came better awareness of structural racism (Lander, 2021). Lockdowns due to COVID-19 were a time when anti-racist activism intensified, and the movement gained more traction. Businesses and public sector bodies alike attempted to incorporate anti-racist messaging and training for their workforce. Unconscious bias training, diversity quotas and publicity were used to claim problems had been addressed and the UK was no longer colour blind. However, as Frankenburg (1993) suggested nearly 30 years ago, colour-blind thinking is exactly that. It embraces diversity while leaving the hierarchies of power unchanged.

Given this context and the fact that colour and racism appear to be more visible now, is colour-blindness still relevant? Critical Race Theory (Delgado and Stefancic, 2017) has in some ways superseded colour-blindness as the lens through which we examine structural racism in society. Critical Race Theory addresses the issue of colour-blindness directly. Despite the rhetoric, colour-blindness remains at the heart of liberalism, with neutrality and equal treatment for all, regardless of personal circumstances or oppression, enshrined in modern law policy and practice (Delgado and Stefancicm 2017). As Delgado and Stefancic suggest:

> If racism is embedded in our thought processes and social structures as deeply as many crits believe, then the 'ordinary business' of society – the routines, practices, and institutions that we rely on to do the world's work – will keep minorities in subordinate positions. Only aggressive, color-conscious efforts to change the way things will do much to ameliorate misery.
>
> (2017: 53)

Societies are not pursuing actively colour-conscious policies in any meaningful way. At an individual level, Bonilla-Silva's research (2018) identifies several personality types that lend themselves to colour-blind thinking, stating that: 'Most whites believe that if blacks and other minorities would just stop thinking about the past, work hard, and complain less (particularly about racial discrimination) then Americans of all hues could "all get along"' (2018: 1). If you were to substitute 'Americans' here for 'British' it would be hard to deny the existence of similar viewpoints expressed on this side of the Atlantic.

The term colour-blindness is not without critics. It is used here as it is the term most commonly referred to in literature. Annamma, Jackson and Morrison (2016) and Frankenburg (1993) suggest, the term colour-evasive is more appropriate. In the phrase colour-blind, 'blindness' is viewed from a deficit model (Annamma, Jackson and Morrison, 2016) and colour-blindness is framed as a passive response. As Frankenburg (1993) argues, being colour-evasive involves purpose, a choice to repress, hide and avoid the reality of systemic racism. (1993: 33).

Systemic racism is a factor in health outcomes for many reasons. Throughout history, trust in the NHS and science more generally among people of colour has been damaged (Geddes, 2021). Breakdown of trust can result in reluctance to access healthcare. People of colour experience a poorer quality of care. The risk of seeking help and not being taken seriously is also a concern. Systemic racism causes minoritised groups to be more likely to fall into lower income brackets and have co-morbidities, increasing health inequalities and COVID risk factors (Geddes, 2021). For Black and Asian pregnant women, one of the risks is less monitoring during pregnancy and hospital stays and a perception they are overreacting to concerns (Kasprzak, 2019). For Black women, the stereotype of the strong Black woman can lead to an assumption of greater ability to endure pain (Graham and Clarke, 2021). Research shows Black women are four times more likely to die in labour than white women, with Asian women twice as likely to die (Kasprzak, 2019). COVID-19 amplified these problems.

For example, Black pregnant women were eight times more likely to be admitted to hospital during the COVID-19 crisis than pregnant white women (NHS England, 2020).

The COVID-19 virus disproportionately affected people of colour (Department of Health and Social Care, 2020). The discourse around the virus was one of the 'great leveller'. Regardless of colour, class or background, it infected anyone at any time. We quickly learned this was not the case.

In June 2020 Public Health England (PHE) published its report *Beyond the Data: Understanding the Impact of COVID-19 on BAME Groups*. The report investigated the raised death rates and more severe symptoms in the Black, Asian and Minority Ethnic (BAME) population, concluding that Black, Asian, and minoritised groups were more likely to live in substandard overcrowded housing, more likely to be employed in frontline jobs with increased exposure to the virus, and more likely to have underlying health conditions due to poverty and stress. BAME communities were also less likely to receive good quality healthcare treatment. Structural inequalities seemed to be at the heart of poorer health outcomes and raised death rates (Public Health England, 2020). At the same time, specific concerns about access to healthcare for undocumented migrants, too afraid to seek healthcare due to the hostile immigration environment, were flagged by charities. The UK mainstream narrative around 'foreigners' and immigration is steeped in racism, and we can see in this example the harm it causes (Bola, 2020).

Stakeholders cited in the PHE report were invited to participate and provide their expertise on how to address issues related to COVID-19. Significantly, they noted the need to address and dismantle structural inequalities in society. For example, it was recommended that employers hire BAME researchers to address current issues and there should be better representation from BAME communities in further research. Action was needed to level the playing field in housing and employment, which contribute to ill health. Trust in healthcare services was highlighted as an issue given the long history of health inequalities among communities of colour. A request was made that the police work with communities to address the increased race hate crime coming from the potential for the portrayal of COVID-19 as a 'BAME disease'. (Public Health England, 2020). Initially Public Health England did not publish any of these recommendations. Kemi Badenoch, Equalities Minister, argued that more data was needed, 'that way we will ensure that we are not taking action that is not warranted by the evidence' (Badenoch, 2020a).

Kemi Badenoch was looking for other types of research to justify action, or inaction, on systemic inequalities in response to COVID-19. Tan (2020) raises the question of power and who determines what *authentic research* is. The world of research has developed within the same society as we all have, where white is the norm, and bias exists, however much we try to discount this (Tan, 2020). Research is commissioned and led predominantly by white males (Woolston, 2020). Given the pervasiveness of colour-blindness in society, further non-stakeholder research would be unlikely to be free from a colour-blind frame of reference. Furthermore, the initial refusal to publish findings implied that there was an attempt to discount, avoid or repress the views of stakeholders (Frankenburg, 1993). This silencing demonstrates how colour-blindness operates in society. The refusal to accept these recommendations as they may not be warranted belies a refusal to see the impact of race discrimination in the crisis.

It took an outcry from the British Medical Association for the recommendations of the PHE report to be published. As Professor Raj Bhopal (2020), a scientist instructed to peer review the stakeholder recommendations, argued: 'If you consult the public, you must publish the results. Otherwise, you've wasted their time, you've wasted your own time, you've wasted taxpayers' money, and you've lost trust' (n.p.). This failure to publish reinforced the lack of trust in healthcare and public services for people of colour and minoritised communities.

Speaking to *The Guardian* in September 2020, Chaand Nagpaul (chair of the British Medical Association) said:

> I am deeply concerned that three months since the publication of the PHE review, we have heard nothing from the government around any specific action or implementation of any of the recommendations. We must remind ourselves that the purpose of the review was to protect a sector of our population who have been disproportionately harmed.
>
> (Nagpaul, 2020: n.p.)

So, were any of the ideas from the Public Health England review taken seriously? Anecdotally there was a broad take up of the idea of risk assessing BAME NHS and social care staff members. If the liberal narrative of society as non-racist and fair permeates management, how would managerial staff assess individual risk and how would a Black or Brown staff member feel at ease in discussing the real issues? The risk assessments were highlighted as an area of concern (Department of Health and Social Care, 2020). Contributors to the BAME Advisory Group report commented on an inertia around risk assessments, suggesting these were only implemented because there was pressure to undertake them. Essentially, risk assessment was seen as a tick-box exercise to cover the employer.

One participant in the BAME Advisory Group research commented: 'White or non BAME colleagues asked about why I was having a workplace risk assessment and not them – it would have been fairer to implement a policy to assess or screen everyone' (n.p.). This quote is an example of the colour-blind liberal discourse described above. It demonstrates a lack of understanding from colleagues as to why minoritised staff would need a differentiated approach due to systemic oppression. Attempts to be colour-conscious here have failed, and the result is a tokenistic gesture leaving staff from affected groups feeling uncomfortable and singled out by the process.

Other examples of colour-blindness in response to COVID-19 can be found in law and order. The systemic racism within the UK police force is well documented (Liberty, 2020). COVID-19 legislation gave increased police powers relating to stop and search and lockdown breach. Police disproportionately targeted Black and Brown individuals, with Black and Brown men 54 per cent more likely to be fined under the coronavirus lockdown powers than white counterparts (Liberty, 2020). We already know the various iterations of stop and search across the decades have been discriminatory. An acknowledgement of the potential for race discrimination in the police response to COVID-19, and a plan to mitigate this was needed. It is not clear if attempts to do this were made, but the statistics show us that, if they were, they were unsuccessful.

At a senior level in policing, colour-blindness continues and structural racism is simply not acknowledged. As the then Metropolitan Police Commissioner Cressida Dick commented 'I don't think we're collectively failing. I don't think [racism] is a massive systemic problem, I don't think it's institutionalised' (Dick, 2020: n.p.). Yet large-scale police discrimination during the COVID-19 crisis has occurred.

Policing during the pandemic has risked the health of people of colour. Netpol's (2020) research found the Black Lives Matter protests were policed in a discriminatory manner and increased the chances of the crowd (including large numbers of Black and Brown people) contracting COVID-19. The report found evidence of 'Kettling, enclosing large numbers of protestors – including children and potentially vulnerable people – in confined spaces for up to eight hours, making social distancing impossible and with no access to toilets, food or water' (Elliot Cooper, 2020: n.p.).

The media narrative characterising these protests as violent was quickly taken up by many to justify police actions, despite the fact most demonstrators were peaceful. Again, colour-blindness played out in this response, demonstrated in the denial and avoidance (Frankenburg, 1993) of addressing any police culpability. Rather than acknowledge the police response was problematic, it was easier to assume that it could not have been, and to view the law as universally fair. Instead, protestors were blamed, both for violence and the spread of COVID-19. I was aware of several Black Lives Matter protests, all of which advised social distancing, mask wearing and hand sanitising. It could be argued that kettling and poor treatment by the police would be more likely to increase transmission.

COVID-19 has highlighted our reluctance to change and acknowledge racism in any meaningful way. It is interesting that Kemi Badenoch, Equalities Minister overseeing this area of policy, openly stands against Critical Race Theory and seems to subscribe to a more colour-blind view herself, casting doubt on the existence for example of white privilege (Badenoch, 2020b: n.p.).

COVID-19 has shone a light on race discrimination, and the Black Lives Matter movement, as well as Critical Race Theory, have made their way into the mainstream. While this is positive, it has also provoked a backlash, seen in the comments of Kemi Badenoch and Cressida Dick. It is clear society pays lip service to race equality while continuing to inflict harm. Are any more focus groups, statistics or stakeholder meetings really needed? The information has been given, repeatedly. The resistance to any meaningful change continues.

Note

[1] For the purposes of this chapter, I have chosen to use the UK spelling of the term 'colour-blind'.

References

Annamma, S.A, Jackson, D.D. and Morrison, D. (2016) 'Conceptualizing color-evasiveness: using dis/ability critical race theory to expand a color-blind racial ideology in education and society', *Race, Ethnicity and Education*, 20(2): 147–162.

Badenoch, K. (2020a) Cited in A. Mohdin, 'Too little date for recommendations in COVID-19 BAME report says minister', *The Guardian*, 4 June [online]. Available from: https://www.theguardian.com/politics/2020/jun/04/too-little-data-for-recommendations-in-COVID-19-bame-report-says-minister

—— (2020b) Cited in A. Woodcock, 'Racism: Equalities minister says anti-discrimination drives can "create a prison for black people"', *Independent*, 28 October [online]. Available from: https://www.independent.co.uk/news/uk/politics/racism-kemi-badenoch-reni-eddo-lodge-critical-race-theory-b1208279.html

Bhopal, R. (2020) Cited in 'BMA demands answers over missing BAME pages of COVID-19 report', *The Guardian*, 13 June [online]. Available from: https://www.theguardian.com/world/2020/jun/13/bma-demands-answers-over-missing-bame-pages-of-COVID-19-report

Bola, G. (2020) 'I'm a public health expert. I know the hostile environment is making the coronavirus outbreak much worse', *Independent*, 13 April [online]. Available from: https://www.independent.co.uk/voices/coronavirus-COVID-19-outbreak-deaths-bame-hostile-environment-immigration-a9462221.html

Bonilla Silva, E. (2018) *Racism Without Racists*, Lanham: Rowman and Littlefield.

Delgado, R. and Stefancic, J. (2017) *Critical Race Theory: An Introduction*, 3rd edn, New York: University Press.

Department of Health and Social Care (2020) 'BAME Communities Advisory Group Report and Recommendations', Gov.uk [online]. Available from: https://www.gov.uk/government/publications/social-care-sector-COVID-19-support-taskforce-report-on-first-phase-of-COVID-19-pandemic/bame-communities-advisory-group-report-and-recommendations

Dick, C. (2020) Cited in A. Forrest, 'Metropolitan Police chief denies force is "Institutionally Racist" and pledges to Listen to Black Lives Matter protestors', *Independent*, 18 July [online]. Available from: https://www.independent.co.uk/news/uk/home-news/met-police-cressida-dick-racism-bianca-williams-stop-search-a9607671.html

Elliot-Cooper, A. (2020) 'Britain is not innocent: a Netpol report on the policing of Black Lives Matter protests in Britain's towns and cities in 2020', *Netpol* [online]. Available from: https://netpol.org/black-lives-matter/

Frankenberg, R. 1993. *White Women, Race Matters*, Minneapolis, MN: University of Minnesota Press.

Geddes, L. (2021) 'COVID Vaccine: 72% of black people unlikely to have jab, UK survey finds', *The Guardian*, 16 January [online]. Available from: https://www.theguardian.com/world/2021/jan/16/COVID-vaccine-black-people-unlikely-COVID-jab-uk

Gotanda, N. 1991. 'A critique of "our constitution is color-blind"', *Stanford Law Review* 44: 1–68. doi: 10.2307/1228940

Graham, R. and Clarke, V. (2021) 'Staying strong: exploring experiences of managing emotional distress for African Caribbean women living in the UK', *Feminism & Psychology*, 31(1): 140–159. doi: 10.1177/0959353520964672

Kasprzak, E. (2019) 'Why are black mothers at more risk of dying', *BBC*, 12 April [online]. Available from: https:www.bbc.co.uk/news/uk-england-47115305

Lander, V. (2021) 'Structural racism: what it is and how it works, *The Conversation*, 30 June [online]. Available from: https://theconversation.com/structural-racism-what-it-is-and-how-it-works-158822

Liberty (2020) 'Pandemic of police powers: Liberty reveals the scale of misuse of police powers under lockdown', *Liberty* [online]. Available from: https://www.libertyhumanrights.org.uk/issue/pandemic-of-police-powers-liberty-reveals-scale-of-misuse-of-police-powers-under-lockdown/

Nagpaul. C. (2020) Cited in 'BMA demands answers over missing BAME pages of COVID-19 report', *The Guardian*, 13 June [online]. Available from: https://www.theguardian.com/world/2020/jun/13/bma-demands-answers-over-missing-bame-pages-of-COVID-19-report

NHS England (2020) *NHS Boosts Support for Pregnant Black and Minority Ethnic Women*, London: NHS England [online]. Available from: https://www.england.nhs.uk/2020/06/nhs-boosts-support-for-pregnant-black-and-ethnic-minority-women/

Public Health England (2020) *Beyond the Data: Understanding the Impact of COVID-19 on BAME Groups*, London: Public Health England [online]. Available from: https://assets.publishing.service.gov.uk/government/uploads/system/uploads/attachment_data/file/892376/COVID_stakeholder_engagement_synthesis_beyond_the_data.pdf

Tan, J. (2020) 'Challenging traditional canons of research' [lecture]. Decolonial Thought and Critical Race Theory, Leeds Beckett University, 1 December.

Woolston, C. (2020) 'White men still dominate in UK academic science', *Nature* [online]. Available from: https://www.nature.com/articles/d41586-020-00759-1

TWELVE

Reviewing the impact of OFQUAL's assessment 'algorithm' on racial inequalities

Bruno Mallett

Introduction

On 20 March 2020, English schools closed indefinitely. This closure lasted five months, only to fully reopen before the next academic year in September 2020. Between May and July, students were commonly expected to sit a series of standardised assessments in primary, secondary, further and higher education institutions. However due to the forced closure of schools, few examinations were taken within schools. Instead, individual grades were estimated through an 'algorithm', a standardised method of assessment prediction based upon a series of metrics that will be discussed later. Centre-assessed grades (teacher predicted grades from this point onwards) was the only recognised alternative to the standardisation algorithm within government, a system that would allow for teachers to predict student outcomes as the formal basis from which final outcomes are drawn. The initial announcement of the algorithm's estimations came on 13 August 2020, the day of the A-level results in England. The results produced widespread inaccuracies, whereby 39 per cent of pupils' grades were 'downgraded' compared to teachers' predictions and previous examination results (Adams, Weale and Barr, 2020). Due to the high-stakes nature of A-levels and the increasing economic and professional importance intricately linked with career opportunities, many students were bemused, and others devastated, at their individual final grades. This individual disappointment collectivised in national protests that attracted significant media attention during the COVID-19 lockdown (Adams and Stewart, 2020; Gant, 2020).

What these protests highlighted was the systemic inequalities in the distribution of attainment levels (Craven, 2020). For example, pupils attending private schools saw the largest attainment 'inflation' in the highest academic accolades, A/A*, when compared with previous years of average institution attainment (OFQUAL, 2020a). Pupils from lower-income, disadvantaged backgrounds suffered the most significant systematic downgrading of results by socioeconomic status (Duncan et al, 2020). Moreover, there were many concerns that the algorithm would also exacerbate existing racialised inequalities in attainment. An Equality and Human Rights Commission report vocalised these concerns, stating that the Office of Qualifications and Examinations Regulation's (OFQUAL)[1] algorithm 'could have a lasting effect on young people from certain ethnic minority backgrounds and disabled pupils and those with special educational needs, who are already disproportionately disadvantaged' if not administered correctly (Wilthew, 2020: 4).

National student-led protests against the use of OFQUAL's assessment algorithm, alongside significant media coverage paid to the protests, successfully pressured the British government to reinstate teacher predicted grades. The algorithm effectively lasted five days, before a 'U-turn' was announced on 17 August 2020 (Weale and Stewart, 2020).

This policy 'U-turn' extended to the awarding of GCSE grades, where students' results were also awarded based upon teacher-predicted grades. In both incidences, there was an average inflation in the results compared to previous years' attainment statistics; a consequence which the government had feared (Baird, 2020). In the aftermath of OFQUAL's algorithm controversy, it inaccurately argued that there was 'no evidence that the process of awarding grades had "introduced bias"' (OFQUAL, 2020b). Although its algorithm did not 'introduce' bias, with regards to creating new socioeconomic paradigms in educational inequality, it exacerbated pre-existing ones. Furthermore, it reflected the permeating function of standardised assessment in global education systems, which perpetuates educational inequality in a myriad of ways, which will be discussed further.

There is a developing plethora of research that focuses on racial attainment gaps across the British education system, which will form the basis of this chapter's central argument in its discussion of the algorithm used by OFQUAL. It is plausible to suggest that the algorithm had significantly widened the attainment gap. In doing so, it remains important to highlight the overall, though statistically nuanced, intersections between racial and economic attainment gaps in the British education system (Strand, 2011).

Critical discussion

Although 38 per cent of students received downgraded results, a percentage of students' grades appeared inflated. Much of the inflation came from the highest grades awarded, namely A/A★ certificates, and mostly from within independent, private institutions (OFQUAL, 2020a). There are many nuances within the inequalities distributed from OFQUAL's algorithm that require further research. However, there are some conclusions that can be drawn from the ways in which it has exacerbated socioeconomic and racial inequalities.

A measurement in OFQUAL's assessment grade prediction included class size as an influencing factor for attainment. It outlined that 'centres with smaller entries will have greater weight placed upon the centre-assessment grades when calculating results, as this is the more reliable source of evidence in these circumstances' (OFQUAL, 2020c: 8). This was initially highlighted as a potential method of comprehensive grade estimation. However, concerns over the validity of results, alongside potential over-inflation caused an initial policy shift towards automated predictors, before the decision was reversed. There is a significant variation of class size depending on the type of institution. Classes that contain a smaller cohort were largely those within private institutions. School sixth forms have an average class size of 11, compared to further education colleges and sixth form colleges, which average 19 students (Parish, Prime and Day, 2017). In private, fee-paying institutions, the average class size narrows beyond that of school sixth forms to an average of 9.4 students per class (Nye and Thomson, 2020a).

A-level subjects that received significant grade inflation among top, A★/A accolades compared with previous attainment, included 'classical subjects' (for example, classical history, history of art and Latin) (Nye and Thomson, 2020b). Classical subjects are rarely available for prospective state college and sixth form students, though are historically synonymous with private forms of education. Although classical subjects did not receive the greatest levels of grade inflation by subject, its inflation symbolised a systematic bias towards private, privileged institutions. Protests against OFQUAL's algorithm throughout August 2020 highlighted this systemic inequality between state and private institutions.

Although there is a similar proportion of students from BAME backgrounds in secondary private institutions in England, 33.8 per cent, compared to state schools, 32.1 per cent (ISC, 2019: 14); ethnicity data for A-level students attending independent institutions is not recorded by the Department for Education census (DfE, 2020). Neither are destinations following studies at independent schools and colleges (DfE, 2019). Investigating racialised inequalities is therefore limited by the gaps in data provided by the Department for Education and other government sources. Although the class size variable inevitably benefits private institutions, more research is required to assess the racial implications of this policy.

Despite limits in available data offered by the Department for Education and OFQUAL, further conclusions can be drawn. For example, another function of OFQUAL's algorithm was to estimate the academic outcome of an individual student through previous attainment statistics of the institution attended. An institution that performs below the national average in its A-level results will affect the awarding of individual results. Students attending these institutions stood a greater risk of receiving downgraded results. The likelihood of Black and minority ethnic students and those from low socioeconomic groups attending such institutions are increased, thus their grades were more likely to be affected. The algorithm used by OFQUAL was a prediction of attainment based upon reflection. For instance, a gap in A-level attainment from consequential socioeconomic impact would require correlating results for the purposes of providing 'validity'. OFQUAL (2020b: 3) summarised its method of estimation as such:

> Standardisation was not solely implemented to ensure that grades were not, overall, excessively high this year. The key purpose was to ensure fairness to students within the 2020 cohort. Without standardisation there was the potential for students to be unfairly advantaged or disadvantaged, depending on the school or college they attended and the approach they took. A key motivation for the design of the approach to standardisation that we took was to remove this potential inequality and, as far as possible, ensure that a grade represents the same standard, irrespective of the school or college they attended.

OFQUAL's argument for 'reducing inequality' is misleading as it does not translate to reducing inequality within pre-existing modes of data. Rather, it confuses 'validity' with 'equality' through the means of achieving statistical similarity. It does not reflect an attempt to narrow attainment gaps. Instead, a review of the emergent discourses on this predominantly argues that the algorithm has exacerbated pre-existing inequalities (Craven, 2020; Duncan et al, 2020). The algorithm intended to produce data which was 'equal' and 'valid,' yet by OFQUALs partial admission, the data produced was merely a reiteration of statistical inequalities in attainment. Data that preceded the automated results of 2020 contain numerous socioeconomic gaps in attainment.

Despite the range of available data on attainment gaps by ethnicity across the education sector in England, including primary, secondary and higher education, only indirect references are made to attainment gaps by ethnicity in further education. For example, in a longitudinal study conducted by the Higher Education Funding Council for England (2018), attainment by ethnicity in further education was used as an independent variable to measure gaps in attainment by ethnicity in higher education. It found that white students, when receiving the same outcomes in further education as Black and other minority ethnic students, were still more likely to achieve better outcomes in higher education. However, this does not measure the differences in attainment by ethnicity in further education. Similarly, in a study sponsored by the then Department for Education and Skills (Connor et al, 2004), the authors could only make broad suggestions on the attainment gaps between ethnic categories in further education, noting that such attainment gaps widened if admitted into higher education due to a number of social, financial and academic factors.

However, some suggestions can be drawn from the data that is available for consideration. Firstly, there is a racialised gap within the enrolment of further education institutions. Some white British students are less likely to pursue formal education post-16 when compared with every minoritised ethnic category. This remains the case, even when similar location and prior GCSE attainment is controlled for (Allan, Parameshwaran and Thomson, 2016). The proportion of students from ethnic minority backgrounds attending further education is 22.6 per cent (ONS, 2020). Though there remains a greater proportion of students from minority ethnic backgrounds attending secondary school, at 29.1 per cent, this can be largely attributed to the increases in pupils from minority ethnic backgrounds entering both primary and secondary educational institutions in England (DfE, 2019). This illuminates the attainment gap that persists between white and minoritised ethnic categories in further education due to the numeric proportion of students at risk of attainment variation.

In addition, there is a validity disparity in the prediction of A-level results, which systematically impacts Black students, as well as other minoritised ethnicities. Everett and Papageourgiou (2011) found that Black students (including Black Caribbean, Black African and Black Other) receive the least accurate predictions of final grade, while white students are the most accurately predicted by racial category. Their research also emphasised that A-level prediction inaccuracy was significant across all ethnic categories. For instance, a recent study by Murphy amd Wyness (2020) found outcome prediction accuracy at around 16 per cent. A common inaccuracy in the prediction of grades is an 'over-prediction' of results achieved by Black students specifically. This can cause negative consequences for pupils as they become 'more likely to apply for more prestigious institutions but then not secure their preferred choice' of university (Bhopal and Myers, 2020). It raises broader questions regarding the ways in which grades are predicted among particular ethnic categories across further education institutions due to the systematic nature of outcome predictions by ethnicity. For example, there remains a lack of ethnic diversity across leadership positions, and staff more broadly, at further education institutions (BFELG, 2020).

Therefore, if Black students are systematically more likely to be 'over-predicted' in their A-level results, OFQUALs decision to install an automated algorithm in the awarding of grades would have likely resulted in a systematic downgrading of A-level results for Black students particularly, though other ethnic minoritised categories would have likely been affected to varying degrees. Instead of the inaccuracies present within teacher-predicted grades, which often represented over-inflated outcomes, the algorithm would have instead reflected significant, pre-existing gaps in attainment between white and all minoritised ethnic categories by design.

Conclusion

Between 13 and 17 August 2020, OFQUAL's distribution of grades based upon a series of numeric estimations was highly controversial. It led to a series of student-organised protests, receiving significant media attention and eventually causing a government U-turn. The systematic downgrading between teacher predicted grades and outcomes produced by the algorithm affected 39 per cent of A-level students. Within these five days, OFQUAL's algorithm was defended by former Education Secretary Gavin Williamson as 'fair and robust' (Sky News, 2020), alongside a report from OFQUAL which summarised that there was 'simply no evidence' of bias in the distribution of results (OFQUAL, 2020b). This conflicted with its own data, which showed significant levels of grade inflation in the highest attainable accolades in private institutions. Smaller classroom cohorts of fewer than 15 students received teacher-predicted grades. This created a disparity between state and private institutions as the former retains much larger classroom cohorts. The average number of students per classroom in private sixth forms is 9.4 (Nye and Thomson, 2020a). There was also a disparity within the downgrading of results when ethnicity and socioeconomic factors were compared. 'Most disadvantaged' pupils were disproportionately affected by downgraded results (Duncan et al, 2020).

This chapter has highlighted a probable racial disparity in the distribution of A-level results. Predictions in A-level results are largely inaccurate, with an accuracy percentage of 16 percent (Murphy amd Wyness, 2020). Predictions for Black students are the 'most inaccurate', while white students receive the most accurately predicted results (Everett and Papageourgiou, 2011). Systematic downgrading between teacher-predicted grades and OFQUAL's algorithm would have likely affected Black students to a much greater extent than white students. This similarly concerns all other racial minoritised ethnic categories, though not likely to the same extent due to the particularly large misprediction of Black students specifically. However, an overall limited amount of available data and research upon attainment and ethnicity in further education limits the conclusion of this study. More research is required to understand the full impact OFQUAL's algorithm and grade distribution of 2020 on Black and other minoritised ethnic students.

Note

[1] The Office of Qualifications and Examinations Regulation (Ofqual) regulates qualifications, examinations and assessments in England: Ofqual – GOV. UK (www.gov.uk).

References

Adams, R. and Stewart, H. (2020) 'Boris Johnson urged to intervene as exam results anger escalates', *The Guardian* [online]. Available from: https://www.theguardian.com/education/2020/aug/16/boris-johnson-urged-to-intervene-as-exam-results-crisis-grows

Adams, R., Weale, S. and Barr, C. (2020) 'A-level results: almost 40% of teacher assessments in England downgraded', *The Guardian* [online]. Available from: https://www.theguardian.com/education/2020/aug/13/almost-40-of-english-students-have-a-level-results-downgraded

Allan, R., Parameshwaran, M. and Thomson, D. (2016) *Social and Ethnic Inequalities in Choice Available and Choices Made at Age 16*, London: Social Mobility Commission.

Baird, J. (2020) 'What are the implications of 2020 grade inflation?', TES [online]. Available from: https://www.tes.com/news/what-are-implications-2020-grade-inflation

Bhopal, K. amd Myers, M. (2020) *The Impact of COVID-19 on A-level Students in England*, Birmingham: University of Birmingham.

Black FE Leadership Group (BFELG) (2020) 'Open letter to address systemic racism in further education', Black Leadership Group [online]. Available from: https://blackleadershipgroup.com/about-us/open-letter/

Craven, J. (2020) *Ofqual Grades Algorithm: A Recipe for Unfairness*, London: upReach.

Connor, H., Tyres, C., Modood, T. and Hillage, J. (2004) *Why the Difference? A Closer Look at Higher Education Minority Ethnic Students and Graduates*, London: HMSO.

Department for Education (DfE) (2019) *Destinations of Key Stage 4 and 16–18 Students, England, 2017/18*, London: HMSO.

—— (2020) 'Students getting 3 A grades or better at A-level', Gov.uk [online]. Available from: https://www.ethnicity-facts-figures.service.gov.uk/education-skills-and-training/a-levels-apprenticeships-further-education/students-aged-16-to-18-achieving-3-a-grades-or-better-at-a-level/latest#by-ethnicity

Duncan, P., McIntyre, N., Storer, R. and Levett, C. (2020) 'Who won and who lost: when A-levels meet the algorithm', *The Guardian* [online]. Available from: https://www.theguardian.com/education/2020/aug/13/who-won-and-who-lost-when-a-levels-meet-the-algorithm

Everett, N. and Papageorgiou, J. (2011) *Investigating the Accuracy of Predicted A-level as Part of 2009 UCAS Admission Process*, London: Department for Business, Innovation & Skills.

Gant, J. (2020) '"Come out Gavin": Hundreds of furious students descend on Westminster for day three of angry protests over A-Level grades chaos as they call for education secretary to be sacked', Daily Mail [online]. Available from: https://www.dailymail.co.uk/news/article-8632239/UK-students-descend-Westminster-day-three-angry-protests.html

Higher Education Funding Council for England (2018) *Differences in Student Outcomes*, London: HMSO.

Independent Schools Council (ISC) (2019) *ISC Census and Annual Report 2019*, London: Independent Schools Council.

Murphy, R. and Wyness, G. (2020) 'Minority report: the impact of predicted grades on university admissions of disadvantaged groups', *CEPEO Working Paper Series 20–07*, London: University College London.

Nye, P. and Thomson, D, (2020a) 'A-Level results 2020: why independent schools have done well out of this year's awarding process', FFT Education Data Lab [online]. Available from: https://ffteducationdatalab.org.uk/2020/08/a-level-results-2020-why-independent-schools-have-done-well-out-of-this-years-awarding-process/

—— (2020b) 'GCSE and A-Level results 2020: How grades have changed in every subject', FFT Education Data Lab [online]. Available from: https://ffteducationdatalab.org.uk/2020/08/gcse-and-a-level-results-2020-how-grades-have-changed-in-every-subject/

OFQUAL (2020a) *Awarding GCSE, AS, A-level, Advanced Extension Awards and Extended Project Qualifications in Summer 2020: Interim Report*, Coventry: OFQUAL.

—— (2020b) *Executive Summary: Awarding GCSE, AS, A-level, Advanced Extension Awards and Extended Project Qualifications in Summer 2020: Interim Report*, Coventry: OFQUAL.

—— (2020c) *Summer 2020 Grades for GCSE, AS and A-level, Extended Project Qualification and Advanced Extension Award in Maths*, Coventry: OFQUAL.

Office for National Statistics (2020) 'Further education participation', Gov.uk [Online]. Available from: https://www.ethnicity-facts-figures.service.gov.uk/education-skills-and-training/a-levels-apprenticeships-further-education/further-education-participation/latest#by-ethnicity-over-time

Parish, N., Prime, V. and Day, S. (2017) *Understanding Costs of A-level Provision via the Decision Making Process Behind Class Sizes*, London: HMSO.

Sky News (2020) 'Education Secretary defends grading system', *YouTube*. Available from: https://www.youtube.com/watch?v=hEU1ba7-ZkY

Strand, S. (2011) 'The limits of social class in explaining ethnic gaps in educational attainment', *British Educational Research Journal*, 37(2): 197–229.

Weale, S. and Stewart, H. (2020) 'A-level and GCSE results in England to be based on teacher assessments in U-turn', *The Guardian* [online]. Available from: https://www.theguardian.com/education/2020/aug/17/a-levels-gcse-results-england-based-teacher-assessments-government-u-turn

Wilthew, A. (2020) *Consultation on an Additional GCSE, AS and A-level Exam Series in Autumn 2020*, London: Equality and Human Rights Commission.

THIRTEEN

The impact of COVID-19 on Somali students' education in the UK: challenges and recommendations

Yusuf Sheikh Omar, Baar Hersi and Abdishakur Tarah

> School closures due to COVID-19 are likely to widen the disadvantage gap.
>
> (Children's Commissioner, 2020)

Introduction

It is estimated there are 300,000–500,000 Somalis in the UK. The Somali community has been present in the UK since the nineteenth century, when Somali seamen settled in Cardiff (Council of Somali Organisations, 2017). The vast majority arrived as refugees after the collapse of the dictatorial regime in early 1991. This led to approximately 16,000 Somalis being granted asylum by 2003 (McCrone et al, 2005).

The unfamiliar community-based UK education system compared to that of Somalia posed enormous challenges to Somali migrants. Such new challenges have been complicated by civil war trauma brought from Somalia, painful experiences in refugee camps before arrival in the UK, and subsequent settlement challenges – social integration, youth identity crises, racism and Islamophobia. These trials have led to emotional difficulties and widespread mental health issues. The combination of these problems has contributed to the Somali community being placed at the bottom of the socioeconomic and educational attainment ladder in the UK.

However, an improvement in Somali students' academic progress has been reported in the last few years before the pandemic (Pells, 2017). The high expectations and investment Somali parents have for their children's education has made a positive impact on outcomes. Similarly, the community tuition centres have contributed enormously to the improvement of Somali children's educational attainment.

Another factor in educational improvement is the common practice among Somali families to enlist the help of community tutors. Furthermore, the cohort of emerging young parents (still a small percentage, but increasing as time passes), who studied in the UK and have a good understanding of the education system and how to support their children's learning, has affected the slow rise in attainment among this community. Unfortunately, COVID-19 brought new challenges that, if not addressed as early as possible, could reverse the progress made possible by this community's hard work.

This chapter discusses how Somali students' educational vulnerabilities were exacerbated by COVID-19. These vulnerabilities stem from existing social inequalities, represented by housing challenges, deprived and impoverished neighbourhoods, socioeconomic issues, unfamiliar educational systems, and poor learning culture within the community. This chapter further explores new challenges brought by the pandemic that have disadvantaged Somali students' learning at home during school closures. It also highlights positive new skills and lessons learnt during school closures, concluding with recommendations.

Methodologies

This chapter is a part of our ongoing research investigating the impact of COVID-19 on the Somali diaspora in the UK. Our first paper (Omar, 2020), published in *African Arguments*, highlighted the vulnerabilities of the Somali diaspora within the pandemic. We employed a triangulation method by combining qualitative and quantitative research methodologies and we conducted semi-structured phone interviews with eight people of Somali origin (two key community leaders, three female schoolteachers, two female parents, and one female school governor). Because of COVID-19 restrictions, we were unable to conduct face-to-face interviews. We also participated in the community online discussions focused on Somali-British community education, which highlighted the effect of the pandemic on student learning processes. Such diverse methodologies validated the findings of our research. The research questions were:

- What are the key challenges encountering Somali-British students during the lockdown caused by COVID-19?
- Can the existing social inequalities disadvantage Somali-British students during school closures?
- What are, if any, the lessons and skills gained during school shutdowns?

Discussion and results

Housing conditions

COVID-19 suddenly changed the logistics of many Somali homes. In intergenerational households, spaces where several individuals may share one room were now makeshift schools and workplaces, making it harder for students to have access to a quiet space for learning (Wallis, 2020). Studies conducted in London in 2017 with 12 Somali boys in year seven (Gillman, 2017) showed that having a quiet space for homework was one of their main challenges. This was reiterated by Ubax, a female primary school teacher in London, who explained in the 'Homeschooling' forum on 10 April 2021 that she experienced, when teaching online, noisy backgrounds caused by crowded quarters and children competing over educational devices. She continued, saying that "we [Somalis] have many children in our houses and it is not easy to buy a device for each child, so they [children] compete who gets the device first".

Kaltuun, a Somali female school governor, shared that some teachers reported that some students from crowded houses preferred to keep their videos off during online learning to avoid any embarrassment if teachers and other students were to witness all the movement in the rooms that they shared with others. As socialisation often occurs through education (Waite and Cook, 2011), a multifamily environment may hinder interactions between teachers and students – disrupting essential social practices of learning environments.

Libraries provided a useful alternative space. For example, Magan, a community leader and an expert in community informal education, argues that before COVID-19 Somali students often visited libraries to study as an alternative to crowded houses. In addition, other social venues such as cafés were used for studying and relaxation purposes. But these facilities were not available due to lockdowns, which in turn affected the students' educational performances. Magan also argued that because Somalis belong to a collectivist rather than individualist cultural background, students learn better with peer friendship groups, which of course was impacted by COVID-19.

Additionally, young people, particularly boys, are physically active and need a space to burn off their energy. In fact, most of the Somali boys we spoke with noted that Physical Education (PE) was one of their favourite lessons. However, PE was not available due to school closures during lockdown and it was near impossible to be physically active in their cramped houses. In relation to this, Bilan, a female teacher –who talked at a Clubhouse Forum entitled 'Somali hour'),[1] observed that students gained weight during school closures due to physical inactivity caused by lack of enough space at home to exercise (Clubhouse, 2021). She also observed that students returned to school in March 2021 with a sense of ambivalence and fatigue caused by living in a deprived environment during school shutdowns.

A similar experience was observed by Mariam Mohamed, a female Somali-American teacher at a school in Minneapolis, USA: 'You have to keep thinking that this child is going through a pandemic, and they're confused and probably bored and stuck at home every day. So, their social-emotional wellbeing is way more important than anything else' (Hersi, 2021). Some educationalists in the UK have expressed the view that a lack of physical activity is highly likely to result in Somali boys under-achieving and perhaps even suffering mental illness (Gillman, 2017). Suffice to say that children who have access to a suitable home learning environment perform better and studied more hours than those living in crowded houses (Sutton Trust, 2020).

Neighbourhood

The effect of living in overcrowded homes is compounded by the poor neighbourhoods where most Somali families live. Since the school closures, around 50 per cent of teachers (Sutton Trust, 2020) at UK state schools in affluent areas reported that they received more than 75 per cent of their students' online homework, compared with 8 per cent of teachers at state schools in poorer and disadvantaged areas. Additionally, around 37 per cent of students from UK state schools in affluent areas already had use of online learning platforms before COVID-19 compared to 23 per cent of students studying at state schools in the deprived areas where the vast majority of Somali students live and study (Sutton Trust, 2020).

Poor life routines

Saharla, a parent, explained that since the school closures children's routines, particularly boys', have deteriorated. She noted that the boys are more likely to play games and may go to bed around 2–3 am. Similarly, Hodan, a Somali female teacher, observed that, in general, Somali students' attendances in online-live lessons were low.

Parents' education

Many Somali parents have limited education and very little or no technological literacy. During COVID-19 they suddenly became makeshift teachers in charge of their children's online learning, a job that even many professionally trained teachers struggled to cope with. This was echoed by Mariam Mohamed from Minneapolis who said:

> The word that comes into my head when I think about this year -with COVID and teaching – is struggle. Technology is really tricky, even for me. I felt like I had to watch a lot of YouTube videos and teach myself before each lesson … So we find ourselves browsing various websites and making purchases that are geared toward online teaching in order to engage and truly educate our students.
>
> (Hersi, 2021)

Somali parents with a low level of digital literacy have been bombarded with information and requests from their child's teachers (Anti-Tribalism Movement, 2020). Online usage can be very harmful (Children's Commissioner, 2020) to students when parents are unable to supervise them properly. The child can simply say, 'I am studying', while possibly engaging in harmful or non-educative online activities. "Boys are on the internet and playing games, all the time, and I don't know what they are doing but they tell me that they are studying", complained Asli, a Somali mother in London, who clearly was aware that such activity would not advance the boys' educational attainment. Since the school closures, over 75 per cent of parents with a postgraduate degree, and just over 60 per cent of those with an undergraduate degree, felt confident in directing their child's learning, compared to fewer than 50 per cent of parents with A-level and GCSE-level qualifications (Sutton Trust, 2020). The percentage is believed to be much lower with parents who have no secondary education. Most middle-aged and older Somali parents fall under the last category, and therefore were unable to support their children's learning.

Despite Somali parents having high expectations for their children (Coughlan, 2017), the limited educational culture in some homes has been detrimental for Somali students' learning since the school closures. "As Somali parents, we are good at telling our children what they should do but we are not good at doing what we are telling them to do … children are more influenced by our actions not words", recounted the teacher Bilan. She suggested that parents should develop a learning culture at home and share it with their children, such as interesting things they have learnt in indirect ways that may resonate with some children and encourage them to learn outside the school context. This would be beneficial to their learning and attainment outcomes. Said Salah (Omar, 2011), who is a prominent teacher of Somali students in Minneapolis, asked his Somali students to count the number of books in their homes and to classify them. The assignment showed that two thirds of Somali families have only a copy of the Quran in Arabic in their homes. Only one third had books other than the Quran. The level of educational performance is often influenced more by the students' home environment than the school in which they study. The internationally renowned sociologist Anthony Giddens found that: 'Children from better-off homes, whose parents take a strong interest in their learning skills and where books are abundant, are more likely to do well in both schools and work than those from homes where these things are lacking' (1993: 862). The lack of a father figure is also a prevalent feature in some Somali households. A father figure is very important particularly for boys' educational and social development in culturally collectivist societies. A significant number of Somali families are run by single mothers (Chorley, 2014). Many of these mothers work as carers and are at home in short sporadic periods. This accords with Mariam Mohamed's observations regarding the Somali community in the US. She said 'Many of the [Somali] parents of the students we work with are essential workers. So, of course, they are not at home during [online] instruction time' (Hersi, 2021).

Somali parents in the UK were heavily reliant on tuition centres and were not necessarily involved directly in their children's learning at home before COVID-19. Many Somali parents consider that their role is to procure their children's tangible educational requirements, such as books, uniforms and food, but then leave it to schools to teach their children. Parents utitlised community tuition centres to help with their child's learning. However, many of these community tuition centres here in the UK were not functioning properly during lockdown, and so there was a lack of access to support resources. This will negatively affect many Somali students' academic attainment and progress.

The vast majority of Somali parents are low-income earners. Since the school closures, high-income parents have shown more satisfaction in their children's online learning than low-income parents. This is probably due to high-income parents' economic capacity to buy the required educational resources; prepare a suitable study environment and engage private online tutors, aspects many low-income Somali parents simply cannot afford. Around 19 per cent of children from middle-class families benefit from £100 or more spending on their education on a weekly basis, compared to 8 per cent in working class families (Sutton Trust, 2020). For instance, three or four Somali children may share one computer at home; socioeconomic circumstances do not allow many families to buy a device for each child. On the other hand, the distribution of the laptops and routers allocated for students from disadvantaged communities like the Somalis was delayed, and that impacted negatively on students' remote learning during school closures (Syal, 2021).

Nevertheless, the Department for Education invested around £2 billion to help students from poor and disadvantaged communities (BBC, 2021); yet Warsame, a managing director of one of the Somali community tuition centres, complained that money went to the established mainstream communities' educational centres, not to marginalised communities. Disadvantaged community tuition centres are struggling. An example of systemic foot-dragging can be found in the fact that £140 million out of the promised £350 million 'Catch Up Fund' for the National Tutoring Programme (NTP) to run across this academic year remained unspent (Whittaker, 2020). Additionally, *The Guardian* unveiled the fact that the 'Catch Up Fund' has not yet reached the most disadvantaged children (Syal, 2021). Meg Hillier, who is the chair of the Commons Public Accounts Committee, confirmed that 'the Department for Education's "failure to do its homework" had hit children who were already most disadvantaged' (BBC, 2021).

In general, the annual 'learning loss' experienced by students from disadvantaged communities during summer time and holidays has already been pronounced. Due to COVID-19, most schools remained closed until September 2020, and the vast majority of students spent around six months out of school since the start of the COVID-19 lockdown on 20 March 2020. That further widened the educational gap between students from disadvantaged backgrounds and those from affluent families (Lander Holloman and Tan, 2021). This was reiterated by Ubax, a primary school teacher in London, who wrote in the Clubhouse forum entitled 'Homeschooling 2021' that, when students returned to school in March, she and other teachers observed a widened gap between students from less-educated and disadvantaged communities and those from well-established families and communities, "Since school closures, many students from disadvantaged ethnic communities like Somalis are far lagging behind and that requires a lot of work to help them catch up others."

Understanding Somali students' emotional challenges caused by school closures

Many Somali families in the UK live in apartments located in high-rise social housing buildings where they can hardly breathe fresh air or find an open space to relax. Staying and studying in such an environment during school shutdowns has caused significant emotional difficulties, stress and mental health issues for Somali children, which undoubtedly negatively impacted their educational achievements. As mentioned before, Magan expressed the view that before the pandemic, going to school, university and public libraries provided many Somali students a convenient learning space, as well a sense of relaxation and peace of mind. However, public venues were not accessible for a long time because of COVID-19. Many Somalians are traditionalist oralists and, therefore, hearing older generations speak about deaths among relatives in the diaspora and back home in Africa has worsened students' emotional suffering, acknowledged Magan.

Many Somali children are facing stressors beyond school examinations (Hersi, 2021). Somali parents, who themselves are stressed and struggling with many life problems posed by the new environment and the virus itself, may not be able to provide enough emotional support for their children. As a young Somali man in London expressed even before the pandemic: 'There is a shortage of emotional intelligence and encouragement in the community' (Omar, 2019).

Misunderstanding of mock exams and students' conditioned behaviourial problems

Magan explains that, back home in Somalia, educational emphasis used to be during the last three to four weeks before the final exam. Magan has observed a cultural continuation within Somali students in the UK. This means that Somali-British students in the UK often increase the intensity of their focus the last few weeks before real exams and, therefore, their educational attainment in the actual exams has been steadily improving. However, both parents and children did not take the mock exams seriously. This is because they anticipated that it was not a real exam and, therefore, would not affect their predicted grades. Warsame recounted the story of a brilliant Somali girl who, before the pandemic, used to be one of the top students in her class. However, because of her misconception about the mock exams, the non-Somali students, who before COVID-19 used to achieve grades lower than her, achieved much better grades than her. This is because these classmates culturally understood the impact of the mock exams on their predicted marks. A social mobility expert has warned that mock exams could have a harmful effect on students from disadvantaged socioeconomic background (Schools Week, 2020).

Warsame explained that Somali families are large in size and households are managed by less-educated single mothers. These resilient and hardworking mothers leave no stone unturned to raise their children in the best way possible in an unfamiliar, complex and culturally diverse society. However, their children, particularly boys aged 12 and above, may exhibit behavioural problems caused by a lack of a father figure. Male role models are essential for boys' growth in culturally collectivist society where stressful housing conditions, deprived neighbourhoods, civil war trauma legacies transmitted through their families and through the wider Somali community can affect their educational development. Similarly, everyday experiences of racism linked to their skin colour, Islamophobia and negative media coverage about Somalis in Africa have perhaps worsened Somali children's behavioural problems. This is compounded by teachers who are unaware and uninformed about the social Somali situation and who do not understand Somali students' extraordinary life challenges and their families' past experiences. A lack of cultural context may lead to negative student–teacher relationships, as well as teachers' negative perceptions of these students. At the end, this may entail teachers' biased assessment against students, explained Warsame.

Skills and experiences gained during school closures

If anything positive can come from the COVID-19 crisis and the subsequent school closures, it has facilitated reconnection, consultation, dialogue and discussion between family members on how to handle their children's education and share overall family tasks. A recent study revealed that, due to COVID-19 lockdowns, many parents, particularly fathers, reported that they 'emerged from this experience more confident as parents and in better relationships with their children' (Vrticka, 2021). Bilan, a primary school teacher, explained that Somali children have also improved their understanding of Somali culture and language skills through everyday interaction with their parents or hearing them speaking over the phones. The home learning system imposed by the pandemic has enhanced parents' understanding of the UK education system and direct involvement in their children's learning process to the point that some families, "have felt that their children can learn better at home than at school", recounted the Somalian teacher Hodan. Furthermore, most teachers who participated in the Clubhouse's 'Homeschooling' community forum on 10 April 2021 agreed that many parents have improved their technological and online skills in order to assist their children. Older siblings have also doubled their efforts to assist their younger siblings' learning at home. However, many older siblings who act as teachers are also students and need to have enough time to study. Such a double task puts enormous pressure on the older siblings, and that may impact negatively on their educational achievements (Hersi, 2021). Interestingly, some families in this study reported the lockdown reduced boys' interaction with peers, including those who could have involved them in drug and criminal activities. At school level, home-based learning has improved teacher–parent constructive communication and collaboration in order to ensure children are on the right track with their learning at home.

Recommendations

To the community

No single solution addresses all the educational challenges faced by Somali heritage youngsters. The authors would urge community professionals in the education sector to organise themselves and discuss the possible ways to support educationally at-risk students and their families. Active Somali community organisations should also advocate at local and national government levels to urge leaders to provide educational resources to vulnerable families and for community tuition centres – a necessary educational provision for the Somali community at this critical time.

To the UK government, Department for Education and schools

We strongly recommend the British government initiate academics to research the short- and long-term impacts of COVID-19 on Somali students' educational attainment and how to improve it. Existing community strengths, as well as the new skills and experiences gained since school closures, should also be appreciated, maintained and reinforced. Different levels of government, including the Department for Education, should provide extra tuition support to students from disadvantaged communities, such as those from refugee and migrant backgrounds like Somalis. The DfE should also monitor the impact of its catch-up arrangements, particularly on disadvantaged children like Somalis, and act on the results. The government and DfE should also provide funding/resources for community tuition centres, which are the backbone for Somali students' educational achievements.

Schools and teachers should understand students' past experiences, the difficulties their families went through, settlement challenges and, therefore, consider these issues when taking key decisions affecting students' long-term life chances, such as mock exams and assessments based-on teachers' predictions. One of the best ways to achieve this is to train teachers on how to understand and respond sensitively to other cultures, with specific emphasis on the cultures of the students populating their particular schools. Another way to fill this gap is to employ educationally trained Somali professionals who can equally understand the mainstream and community cultures and, therefore, are able to bridge the gap, reconcile cultural differences and liaise between the outcomes of Somali community/students of Somali heritage on the one side and schools/teachers on the other side.

Note

[1] The Clubhouse 'Somali hour forum' is a weekly online Somali-British community platform organised every Saturday at 6pm. The main aim of this forum is to facilitate the Somali-British community to discuss and understand pressing issues facing the community, including the UK education system and the challenges facing their children, in order to help them improve their children's learning culture.

References

Anti-Tribalism Movement (2020) 'COVID-19 in the Somali community: urgent briefing for policy makers in the UK' [online]. Available from: https://theatm.org/wp-content/uploads/2020/04/COVID-19-Impact-on-the-Somali-Community-ATM-2020.pdf

BBC (2021) 'COVID: Catch-up tuition not helping poorest pupils, says NAO', BBC, 17 March [online]. Available from: https://www.bbc.co.uk/news/education-56418905

Chorley, M. (2014) 'Which ethnic group is still most in love in marriage? (Clue – They are not in British-born)', *Daily Mail*, 24 June [online]. Available from: https://www.dailymail.co.uk/news/article-2666908/British-families-likely-tied-knot-moved-India-Sri-Lanka-Afghanistan.html

Children's Commissioner (2020) 'Briefing: tackling the disadvantage gap during the COVID 19 crisis', *Children's Commissioner*, 22 April [online]. Available from: https://www.childrenscommissioner.gov.uk/report/tackling-the-disadvantage-gap-during-the-COVID-19-crisis/

Clubhouse (2021) 'Somali hour', *Clubhouse* [online]. Available from: https://www.clubhouse.com/club/SomaliHour

Coughlan, S. (2017) 'Migrants have raised school standards in London, says Gove', BBC, 18 March [online]. Available from: https://www.bbc.co.uk/news/education-39285039

Council of Somali Organisations (2017) 'Somalis and mental health: raising awareness and developing interventions that improve outcomes', *Council of Somali Organisations* [online]. Available from: https://www.councilofsomaliorgs.com/sites/default/files/resources/CSO-M.Health%20Report.pdf

Giddens, A. (1993) *Sociology*, London: Blackwell Publishers.

Gillman, P. (2017) 'The achievement of Somali boys: a case-study in an inner-London comprehensive school', MSc thesis, University of Oxford.

Hersi, B. (2021) 'Minneapolis teacher Mariam Mohamed thinks the emotional health of her students is more important this year than their multiplication tables', *Sahan Journal*, 13 January [online]. Available from: https://sahanjournal.com/stories-from-the-pandemic/minneapolis-teacher-mariam-mohamed-COVID-19/

Lander, V., Holloman, T.R. and Tan, J. (2021) 'Collaboratives on addressing racial inequality in COVID recovery: education, a briefing paper, collaboratives on addressing racial inequality in COVID recovery', London. doi: 10.1111/j.1468-0319.1985.tb00102.x

McCrone, P., Bhui, K., Craig, T., Mohamud, S., Warfa, N., Stansfeld, S., Thornicroft, G. and Curtis, S. (2005) 'Mental health needs, service use and costs among Somali refugees in the UK', *Acta Psychiatrica Scandinavica*, 111(5): 351–357.

Omar, Y. (2011) 'Integration from youth perspectives: a comparative study of young Somali men in Melbourne and Minneapolis', PhD thesis, La Trobe University, School of Social Sciences.

—— (2019) 'Young Somali men growing up in the west left alienated and at risk of violence', *The Conversation* [online]. Available from: https://theconversation.com/young-somali-men-growing-up-in-the-west-left-alienated-and-at-risk-of-violence-106664

—— (2020) 'Why is the Somali diaspora so badly hit by COVID-19?', African Arguments, 13 May [online]. Available from: https://africanarguments.org/2020/05/13/why-is-the-somali-diaspora-so-badly-hit-by-COVID-19/

Pells, R. (2017) 'Michael Gove: immigrant children improve results and drive up school standards', *Independent*, 17 March [online]. Available from: https://www.independent.co.uk/news/education/education-news/immigrant-children-improve-results-drive-up-school-standards-education-michael-gove-london-dubai-a7637206.html

Schools Week (2020) 'Using mock exams as 'back-ups' could 'compound' disadvantage', *Schools Week*, 3 November [online]. Available from: https://schoolsweek.co.uk/using-mock-exams-as-back-ups-could-compound-disadvantage/

Sutton Trust (2020) 'COVID 19 and social mobility: impact brief #1: school shutdown', *Sutton Trust*, April [online]. Available from: https://www.suttontrust.com/wp-content/uploads/2020/04/COVID-19-Impact-Brief-School-Shutdown.pdf

Syal, R. (2021) 'Schools COVID catch-up programme "not reaching disadvantaged pupils"', *The Guardian,* 17 March [online]. Available from: https://www.theguardian.com/world/2021/mar/17/schools-COVID-catch-up-programme-not-reaching-disadvantaged-pupils

Vrticka, P. (2021) 'Caring, confident dads have structurally different brains – new research', *The Conversation* [online]. Available at: https://theconversation.com/caring-confident-dads-have-structurally-different-brains-new-research-171137

Waite, L. and Cook, J. (2011) 'Belonging among diasporic African communities in the UK: plurilocal homes and simultaneity of place attachments', *Emotion, Space and Society*, 4(4): 239.

Wallis, W. (2020) 'How Somalis in East London were hit by the pandemic', *Financial Times*, 22 June [online]. Available from: https://www.ft.com/content/aaa2c3cd-eea6-4cfa-a918-9eb7d1c230f4

Whittaker, F. (2020) 'Government "misled" school leaders over National Tutoring Programme cash', *Schools Week*, 4 December [online]. Available from: https://schoolsweek.co.uk/government-misled-school-leaders-over-national-tutoring-programme-cash/

Conclusion: Long COVID, long racism

Whether denied, derided or determined to overcome it, COVID-19 has impacted many lives in ways that we are only now beginning to witness, as we move from old configurations of normality and adapt to new realities, be it flexible ways of working and learning or working to change social systems. It is also evident that COVID-19 extends beyond a global health problem. Sociocultural readings of the pandemic have pointed to this as a crisis on multiple levels – economic, environmental, social, cultural and racial. It, then, becomes an important task to understand how this crisis has affected, and continues to affect, people across the world, through readings that do not lean into othering and moralism, as is often the main societal response, and as we have seen throughout this text.

With no end yet in sight, COVID-19 and its variants – from the South African variant to Omicron then to Omicron BA.4 to BA.5 – are still widespread and affecting the lives and health of many people. And amid the political and social turmoil of summer 2022, as the populace contends with strikes by railway workers and barristers, the cost of living crisis and the political turbulences of the British government, we must remember and be ever vigilant of the impact of the rampant racism evident in our society. In the early days of the pandemic, the COVID variants were not referred to by scientific nomenclature but by the site of origin – for example COVID-19's origins in China, then the South African strain, then the Indian strain. This associated racialisation of a virus was intriguing to observe, since it resurrected and reinforced the trope of dirty unclean foreigner/outsider/subaltern, and drew implicit links between biology and race. The naming of the variants by country of origin was eventually dropped in favour of scientific nomenclature. This may have occurred as someone, somewhere, realised that the links between the easy and lazy association of the new variant by country of origin could reinforce certain racial stereotypes. But the damage had already been done. So, while at the same time living with and suffering from the virus, Black and global majority people have suffered insulting microaggressions associated with the early identification of the COVID-19 virus variants, and simultaneously been lost to the virus in greater numbers. The saying 'adding insult to injury' jumps to mind.

In the background, the spectre of racism and its effects have continued unabated. The intimate strip search of a Black female student (Child Q) in secondary school by London's Metropolitan Police Service in 2020 is rooted in privilege, presumptions, and power. The 2022 report of the Child Q case illustrates not only normalised adultification of Black youngsters but also the race ignorance that prevails among educational, health and law enforcement professionals. Since 2020 there have been numerous accounts in the media of racism, from the racial abuse suffered by the three Black England footballers at Euro 2020, the years of racist abuse suffered by Azeem Rafiq at Yorkshire County Cricket Club, to the report produced by Health Education England in March 2022 on the experience of racial discrimination and harassment in London primary care. Just as COVID-19 casts a shadow over the lives of those inflicted with long COVID, the pall of racism blights the lives and lived experience of people of colour. While science will keep pace with the COVID-19 virus by designing annual vaccines to ensure we do not endure another COVID pandemic, the historical and contemporary pandemic of racism appears to run rampant in the absence of inoculation. It mutates and infects, leaving casualties in its wake. What does this mean for anti-racism? For years, those on the frontlines of anti-racism have pleaded with the same governments in existence today to help eradicate the disease of racism. Monies, research and mandates have poured into the pandemic of racism just as they have for COVID-19. Yet, racism appears never-ending. It is quite unsettling to realise how we can easily envision the end of the COVID-19 pandemic (and the return of 'normality'), but can scarcely conjure an image of an anti-racist world. With that in mind, the authors in this collection bring forth their stories, as countering majoritarian narratives, and through a critical race lens.

Each chapter is a different story, tied together by the known and unknown effects of COVID-19, yet with the overwhelming awareness of the materiality of racism. Authors representing a variety of geographies, languages, faiths and pursuits offer a down-to-earth analysis of their views of these colliding pandemics. The collection opened with the blame culture that often follows the othered BAME around, moved to the intersection of Britain's honours system, with not only Black Lives Matter but also the government's COVID-19 response, and then moved to Black vaccination hesitancy in the US and the racialised closure of Historically Black Colleges and University (HBCU) medical schools. The discussion then spotlighted the experience of being a Black millennial expectant mother amid the pandemic and protests, the resurrection of race science and waves of anti-Asian hate, and the exacerbation of the green space gap and racialised access to recreational cricket for South Asian communities. We turned our attention to the challenging burial rites and bereavement experienced by British Bangladeshis, interrogating the progress, problems and potential of racial justice and equalities law, and deeply reflecting on the disproportionality of who gets to breathe. Following this, we explored the label BAME and the effect of this usage on identity within the coronavirus context, and the paradox of racism and colour-blindness in the Metropolitan Police and National Health Service. We drew to a close by reviewing the impact of OFQUAL's assessment algorithm on racial inequalities and with a discussion of Somali students' educational vulnerabilities, exacerbated by COVID-19. Finally, the effects of long COVID are continuously being learned, as COVID-19 itself is still changing.

This collection does not seek to offer a totalising version of Black and global majority lived experiences of COVID-19. There are limitations to this piece – for example the absence of the voices of Uber drivers, small business owners, or cleaning staff, just to give a few examples. What we hope we have The chapters in this collection shine a light on the importance of acknowledging the sociocultural contexts of COVID-19 experiences through a critical race lens, and also their affective, temporal and spatial dimensions. In the first wave of the pandemic, we learnt that conditions are subject to swift change, and that complacency or reactive decision-making, rather than proactively considering long-term and inclusive solutions to mitigate the multidimensional effects of the mutating virus, can have damaging effects. As we enter into the next stages of the pandemic, it becomes an important endeavour to develop and maintain critical, anti-racist, decolonial and intersectional approaches that acknowledge the complexities and effects of diverse lived experiences in a long-COVID society, and one where care is at the heart of human relations.

Index

A

AAME *see* African, Asian and Minority Ethnic (AAME)
abortion and infanticide 39
academic prestige hierarchy (APH) 38, 42–3, 47–8
adverse childhood experiences (ACEs) 135–6
African, Asian and Minority Ethnic (AAME) 160
African Arguments 201
Afriphobia 164
aggressive behavior 164
Aguirre, A. 83
Aldridge, A.W. 159
A-level attainment 191
A-level prediction inaccuracy 193
Allen, A. 61
All-Party parliamentary group (APPG) 136–7
AMA *see* American Medical Association (AMA)
American Medical Association (AMA) 45–6, 49
angry Black woman 66
animal-to-human transmissions 85
Annamma, S.A. 178
antagonism 1
anti-Asian
  hate crimes 4, 218
  immigration laws 80
  racism 76–9, 85
anti-BAME 161
anti-Chinese/Asian racism 76–9, 84
anti-colonial arguments 29
anti-colonial uprisings 18
anti-immigration stance 81
anti-racism/racist 19, 26–7, 29, 79, 103
  activism 177
  statements 15
  uprising 10–11
anxiety and insecurity 132
Anyiam, S. 4
APH *see* academic prestige hierarchy (APH)
APPG *see* all-party parliamentary group (APPG)
Aspinall, P.J. 160, 163
Atherton, F. 15
attainment gap 8, 193
Australian racial 47
auto-ethnographies 16–17, 60
awareness 154

B

'bad death' 114–15
Badenoch, K. 180, 183
BAME *see* Black, Asian or minority ethnic (BAME)
BAME Advisory Group report and research 181
#BAMEOver 169
Bangladeshi community 118, 121–3. *see also* Muslim funerals
Bangladeshi-heritage people 110
Bell, J. 46
Belong Here (2021) 102

INDEX

Best, S. 85
Beyond A Boundary (1963) 100
Bhopal, R. 180
BIMA *see* British Islamic Medical Association (BIMA)
biodiversity loss 83
Blacks
  achievement 19–20
  and Brown people voices 38
  communities 162
  and global majority communities 4
  healthcare 3
  inferiority 38, 39–42
  medical professionals, threat of 44–5
  millennial resistance 4, 59
  people, life expectancy 52
  resistance 66
  reticence 3
  students, predictions for 195
Black, Asian or minority ethnic (BAME) 6–7, 10–12, 91–2, 157–69
  communities 4, 158
  mortality rates 10
  non-European heritage 158
  people who experience racism/PoWER 169
  racial frustrations 11
  racially minoritised 168–9
  in UK government 158
Black and Minority Ethnic (BME) 160
Black British Academics 168
(Black) British Empire 28–9
Black Lives Matter (BLM) 3, 4, 16–17, 27, 67, 177
  activism 10–11
  movement 164, 183
  protests 59
#BlackPoWER 169
Black-racialised man 3
Black Skin, White Masks (1952) 20
Black vaccination reticence
  academic prestige hierarchy (APH) 42–3
  American Medical Association (AMA) 45–6
  Black inferiority 39–42
  Black medical professionals, threat of 44–5
  Carnegie Foundation influence 46–8
  Critical Race lens 38–9
  Flexner, A. 3, 37–8, 48–52
  HBCU medical schools, Flexner impact 50–1
  Healthcare repercussions 51–2
  land-grant colleges and universities 43–4
  models of exclusion 45
Blair, T. 26
BLM *see* Black Lives Matter (BLM)
BLM international protest 61
Bohm, D. 155
Bolly Cric-Hit 98
Bonilla Silva, E. 177–8
Bovine Spongiform Encephalopathy (BSE) 85
Braidotti, R. 151
breathing
  difficulty, death 114–15
  space 149
Bristol City Council 139
British anti-racism 17
British–Bangladeshi community 5, 112. *see also* Muslim funerals
British Black Lives Matter 15
British education system 189
British government, political turbulences 216–17
British Islamic Medical Association (BIMA) 114, 117
British Muslim community 92
British–Muslims' funeral needs 111–13
British Natural History Museum 76
Britishness 165
Brown, D. 60

C

CALC (Compassion, Accuracy, Linguistic, Context) 159
Cameron, David 131–2

Campaign to Protect Rural England (CPRE) 101
capitalism 24–5, 83, 151
capitalist society 16
Carnegie, A. 40, 47
Carnegie Foundation for the Advancement of Teaching (CFAT) 47, 49–50
Carnegie Foundation influence 46–8
Carnegie Institution of Washington 40–1
Carrington, B. 96
Case Western University 47
Caucasian persuasion 25–8
celebrity activism 28
centrality of racism 38
centre-assessed grades 187–8
Centre for Race, Education and Decoloniality (CRED) 2
Chadha, G. 101
Chave, A. 97–8
Chinese–Asian communities 72
Chinese virus 2, 84
Civil Rights Movement 38, 45
Civil War recovery 41–2
Clarke, B. 61
collective unconscious 165
colonialism 16, 100, 154
colonial services 21
colour-blindness concept 7, 176–7
  liberal discourse 181–2
  racism 7, 62, 166
  racist society 67
colour-conscious policies 177–8
colour-evasive 178
Colston, E. 141
Commission for Equality and Human Rights 130
Commission for Racial Equality (CRE) 130
commodification of Blackness 154, 166
Commonwealth immigrants 110–12
community-based insurance scheme 122
community tuition centres 206
community tutors 200

Compassionate, Accurate, Linguistically sound and Contextually conscious (CALC) 6–7
confusion, psychiatric symptoms 163–4
convergence of interest 38
Council on Medical Education of the AMA 49
Countryfile 105
COVID-1984 14–30
cricket 4, 5, 91–100, 104–5, 218
Critical Race lens 38–9
Critical Race Studies 2
Critical Race Theory (CRT) 3, 38, 66, 177, 183
critique of liberalism 38
CRT *see* Critical Race Theory (CRT)
cultural and organisational change 104
cultural resonance 71
culture clash model 96–7

D

Darlington- Pollock, F. 136–7
Data Protection Act 2018 114
Dattani, N. 97
Davis, A. 150
death
  'bad death' 114–15
  breathing difficulty 114–15
  certificate 116–17
  dead body washing and shrouding, regulations on 117–18
  in minority ethnic groups 159
  psychological distress 114–15
  social isolation 114–15
decolonisation 152, 154
Delgado, R. 177
Democratic Republic of the Congo 151
Department for Health (DfH) 75
depression 163–4
Detzler, M. 79
Dick, C. 182
digital activism 99
digital literacy 204–5
disability 131–2

INDEX

Disability Rights Commission (DRC) 130
discrimination and prejudice 1
discriminatory policies and Black community tools 38
disenfranchisement and domestic terrorism 45
diversity 22, 28
Doharty, N. 66
Dorrell, S. 85
Dream Big Desi Women campaign, 2021 98
dual citizenship 111
Duggan, M. 61
dying in isolation with no spiritual support 114–16

E

ecotherapy 90
educational culture 205
educational inequality 189
educational performance level 205–6
Eliot, C. 47
emotional intelligence 208
empathy 140–1
Empire's Child (2021) 27
empowerment 94
encouragement in community 208
equalities, socio-economic clause in 134–5
Equalities Bill 131–2
Equality Act 132–3
Equality Act 2010 5, 129, 136, 138–9, 141
Equality and Human Rights Commission 130, 139, 188
Equal Opportunities Commission (EOC) 130
ethnic 165
  children 165
  ethnicity data for A-level students 190–1
  minority 23, 164
  practice 154–5
  teachers 165
ethno-religious groups 96
Eugenic Record Office (ERO) 40, 44
eugenics 12, 40–3

Eurocentric colonial attitudes 168
European immigrants with Bangladeshi ancestry 111
European imperialism and colonialism 148
Evans, G. 82
Everett, N. 193

F

Fairer Scotland Duty 138
Fanon, F. 20, 161, 165
father figure, in educational and social development 206
Fletcher, T. 96
Flexner, A. 3, 37–8, 48–52
Floyd, G. 15, 26–7, 64, 66, 81, 146, 151
forest bathing 90
Fowler, C. 102
Frankenburg 178
Freire, P. 152
frontline jobs 110–11
funeral rites 109–10

G

Gates, B. 123
#GayPoWER 169
gender
  inequalities 97
  pay gap 90
  and race equality 130, 132
General Data Protection Regulation (UK GDPR) 114
ghusl practice 117
Giddens, A. 205–6
Glover Report (2019) 102
grade prediction 190
(green) parks and recreation
  community-centred approach 102
  costs and accessibility 101
  deprivation 90
  green space gap 90–1
  health and wellbeing 101–3
  material urbanism 101
  mischaracterisation 102
  personal pandemic postscript 103–5

racial and social injustice 98–9
space gap 90–1
unequal by design 91–3
Green Space Index 89
grief and mourning expression 112
Guardian, The 133, 181
Gypsies 163

H

Hancock, M. 75
Hancock, S. 61
Harman, H. 133
Harriman, M.W. 40
health
 disparities 136–7
 inequalities 90, 163, 178–9
Healthcare repercussions 51–2
healthiness 149
hereditary aristocracy 18
Hiatt, M.D. 49
Higher Education Funding Council for England (2018) 192
Hillier, M. 207
Hinchcliffe, J. 7
Historically Black College and University (HBCU) medical schools 38, 50–1, 218
Holloman, T.R. 3
home-based learning system 210–11
home-based office 73
Honours system 3, 26, 29
Huanan Market, Wuhan 84
human
 rights violators 15
 trafficking of Black people 19
Hunter, S. 22
hypercriminalisation of Black youth 61
hypervisibility of Blackness 66

I

immunisation 148
inclusion 150
income and race 90
index of multiple deprivation (IMD) 136

Indian and Black Caribbean people deaths 159
Indian variant 2
Indigenous communities 155
inequalities 1, 15, 89, 138, 189–90
inequities 149
informal education 202
informed consent 113–14
inherited cerebral matter 165
institutionalised racism 81
institutional racism 4, 61
institutional rejection 99
institutional violence 27
institutional whiteness 28
international BLM protests 62
International Monetary Fund, 2020 90
intersectionality 163
intersections of inequality
 education and activism 151–5
 right to breathe 147–51
Islam, F. 5
Islamic funeral rites in UK 111–12
Islamic mourning practices 120–1
Islamophobia and racism 200

J

Jackson, D.D. 178
James, C.L.R. 100
Janazah 119–20
Johnson, B. 75, 93
Jukes, P. 25–6
Jumbe, S. 159

K

'*kalema*' 115
Kay, K. 4–5
Kidambi, P. 93
Kinouani, G. 20
Kitchener, L. 21
Klingberg, T. 83, 84

L

labour legislation 90
'land-grab universities' 43

INDEX

land-grant colleges and universities 43–4
language barriers 115
LBN *see* left-behind neighbourhood (LBN)
learning
 home-based 210–11
 loss 207
 space 208
Leeds Beckett University 2
left-behind neighbourhood (LBN) 136–8, 141–2
leisure under lockdown 92
Lentin, A. 153
Leong, N. 23–4
Lescure, R. 161
libraries 202
London Cricket Trust 100–1
London Writing Guy 95
Lorde, A. 165–6
low-income earners 206

M

Macdonald, I. 96
Mallett, B. 7–8
Manzoor-Khan, S. 20, 150
Martin, G. 29
material urbanism 101
meritocracy 149
Mill, J.S. 154–5
Milner, A. 159
minoritised communities 180
Minority Ethnic 164
minority/minorities 165, 168
mischaracterisation 102
mixed heritage perspective 4
mock exams, impact 209
models of exclusion 45
Mohamed, M. 203, 204
Monbiot, G. 21
morbidity 1
Morrill Acts 43, 47
Morrison, D. 178
mortality 1
Morton, S.G. 46
Moshie-Moses, I. 6–7
Mott, L. 136–7
multifamily environment 202
Munford, L. 136–7

Murphy, R. 193
Muslim funerals
 British–Muslims' funeral needs 111–13
 costs 118
 dead body washing and shrouding, regulations 117–18
 dying in isolation with no spiritual support 114–16
 funeral rites 109–10
 future practice, recommendations for 121–3
 grief and mourning expression 112
 Islamic funeral rites in UK 111–12
 methodology 113–14
 socially distanced funeral prayer *(Janazah)* 119–20
 socially distanced mourning 120–1
 waiting time 116–17
myth of return 111–12

N

Nagpaul, C. 181
National Burial Council 114, 117
National Health Service (NHS) 17
national instability from immigration 41
National student-led protests 188–9
National Tutoring Programme (NTP) 207
Native American property 43
nativist counterattack 42
Natural Greenspace Standards 91
Nenequirer, The 19
neutrality crops 148
Noah, T. 23
non-European heritage, BAME 158

O

Office of Qualifications and Examinations Regulation (OFQUAL) assessment algorithm 8, 187–95
 A-level attainment 191

attainment gap 193
Black students, predictions for 195
British education system 189
centre-assessed grades 187–8
classical subjects 190
educational inequality 189
ethnicity data for A-level students 190–1
grade prediction 190
inequalities 189–90
National student-led protests 188–9
pre-existing gaps 194
racial disparity 195
racialised gap 192–3
racialised inequalities 191, 219
standardisation 191
systematic inequalities 188
teacher-predicted grades 194
O'Gaunt, J. 75
Omar, Y.S. 8
Omicron 216
one-size-fits-all method 162
online homework 203
Operation Legacy 25
Order of the British Empire (OBE) 16

P

pandemic 1
Papageourgiou, J. 193
Payne, G. 165
pedagogy 152–3
People Of Colour (POC) 162–3, 180
personality, colour-blind thinking 178
personal pandemic postscript 103–5
perspectives of intersectionality 38
Pew Research study 37–8
Phan, P.H. 83
PHE *see* Public Health England (PHE)
physical discomfort 114–15
Physical Education (PE) 202–3
POC *see* People Of Colour (POC)

postcolonial banter 19–25
'post-race' society 166
poverty and stress 179
PoWER 169
pregnancy
  auto-ethnographic entry 62–5
  Black women and infants, mortality rates 65–6
  experiencing 62–3
  invisibility and silencing 66
  post-pregnancy and during protest 63–5
Pritchett, H.S. 48–9
Progressive Era liberal policies 39
PSED *see* Public Sector Equality Duty (PSED)
psychological distress, death 114–15
public discourse 176–7
Public Health England (PHE) 75, 110, 179
Public Sector Equality Duty (PSED) 135, 139
Puwar, N. 92–3

R

race/racial
  attainment gaps 8
  -based immigration quotas 41
  capitalism 23–4
  discourse 168
  discrimination 52, 66, 163, 178, 183
  disparity 169, 195
  educational attainment, gaps in 90
  frustrations 11
  gap 192–3
  genealogy of cricket 96–7
  hierarchy 45
  and identity 90
  ignorance 217
  inequalities 6, 191, 219
  injustices 162
  language 6–7
  minorities 168
  minoritised 168–9
  pedagogy 60
  segregation 47

INDEX

and social injustice 98–9
suicide 46–7
superiority 1
racial justice and equalities law 218
  2010–2020 131–9
  culture wars 139–41
Racial Justice Network 60
racism 19, 151, 152–3, 165–6
  in Britain 62
  Chinese community 77–8
  colonialism and 91
  criminalisation and 62
  Islamophobia and 200
  processes 139–40
racist ideology 46
Rafiq, A. 94, 217
Ratna, A. 95
recreational cricket 99
respectability 20, 27–8
resurrection of race science
  anti-Asian racism 76–81
  pandemic and racism 72–6
  zoonotics, virological origins and science of blame 81–4
Richardson, R. 5, 161, 164, 165
'right to say goodbye' 115
Rodney, W. 24
Romani people 163
Roosevelt, T. 46–7
Roy, A. 142
Rural Racism (2004) 102
Ryder, M. 169

S

Saini, A. 82
Sakar, A. 28
Sanghera, S. 93
SARS-Cov-2 (COVID-19) 1, 86
scientific-appearing aggregational hierarchy 41
Scottish Muslim Funeral Services 119
Sethi, A. 102
Shiva, V. 103
Sidhu, H. 95, 97–8
Sidhu, J. 166
Siler-Holloman, L.A. 3
Simone, N. 16

slave emancipation 41–2
slave-trader 141
Smith, G. 15, 83
Smith, L.T. 148
Soames, N. 16
social capital 47
social determinants of health 134
social-emotional wellbeing 203
social integration 200
socialism 133
social isolation, death 114–15
social justice power 38
socially distanced funeral prayer (*Janazah*) 119–20
socially distanced mourning 120–1
social mobility 209
social reality 7
socio-economic disadvantage 133
socio-economic inequalities 139
Somali-British community education 201
Somali students' education in UK
  to community 211
  community-based UK education system 199–200
  emotional challenges 208–10
  housing conditions 201–3
  life routines 204
  methodologies 201
  neighbourhood 203
  parents' education 204–8
  skills and experiences gained 210–11
  tuition centres 200
  UK government, Department for Education and schools 211–12
  vulnerabilities 200
South Asian Action Plan, 2018 104
South–Asian ancestry 109–10
South Asian communities 4–5
space invaders 96
spiritual end-of-life support 115
Sport England (2015) 101–2
standardised mortality ratios (SMR) 159
Stefancic, J. 177

Stelling, J. 26
stigmatisation fear 121
Stone, C.T. 19
stress 136
stress and anxiety 163–4
structural inequalities 147, 179
structural racism concept 2, 139–40, 177, 182
Subjection of Women, The 154–5
systemic inequalities 180, 188
systemic racism 178–9
Sze, S. 159

T

TAOBQ *see* The African Or Black Question (TAOBQ)
Tate, S.A. 66
tayammum (dry washing) 117
teacher-parent constructive communication 211
teacher-predicted grades 194
teachers' biased assessment 210
The African Or Black Question (TAOBQ) 160
therapeutic practice 153
thinking of identity 161
Thwing, C.F. 47
transatlantic slave trade 40
Travellers 163
Trump, D. 81
Truss, L. 140
trust, healthcare services 179–80
Tuskegee Study 148

U

UK, COVID-19 176–83
UK Social Research Association ethical guidelines 114
unconscious bias training 177
utilitarianism 155

V

vaccine misinformation 38
value-judgment rankings 40–1
video conferencing and funeral 119–20
vindication 94
virus of racism 1

W

waiting time, Muslim funerals 116–17
Wang, S. 79
wealth accumulation 47
Westerners 161
White, C. 27
whiteness 38, 42–3, 149
whiteness as property 38, 42
white supremacy 3, 60, 165
Whitty, C. 15
Williams, P. 61
Williamson, G. 194
Wilson, W. 47
#WomanPoWER 169
Wood, G. 83
Wretched of the Earth, The (2001) 154
Wuhan 70, 71, 75, 80, 84
Wyness, G. 193

Y

Yep, G.A. 161
Yorkshire County Cricket Club 94, 217
youth identity crises 200
YouTube videos 204
Yusuf, H. 150

Z

Zephaniah, B. 29, 101
zoonotics, virological origins and science of blame 81–4